THE SOLUTION TO
BACK AND NECK PAIN
That No One is Telling You About

THE SOLUTION TO BACK AND NECK PAIN

That No One is Telling You About

Dr. Ben Grams, D.C.

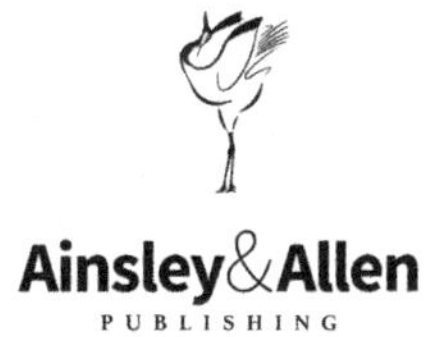

Ainsley & Allen Publishing LLC

ISBN: 978-0-9983503-0-1

First Printing 2016

20 19 18 17 16 5 4 3 2 1

Edited by Connie Anderson, Words & Deeds, Inc.
Cover photo and design by Amp 13 Graphic Design
Interior design by Sue Stein

The Solution to Back and Neck Pain That No One is Telling You About is a work of nonfiction. The names, details, and circumstances have been changed to protect identities.

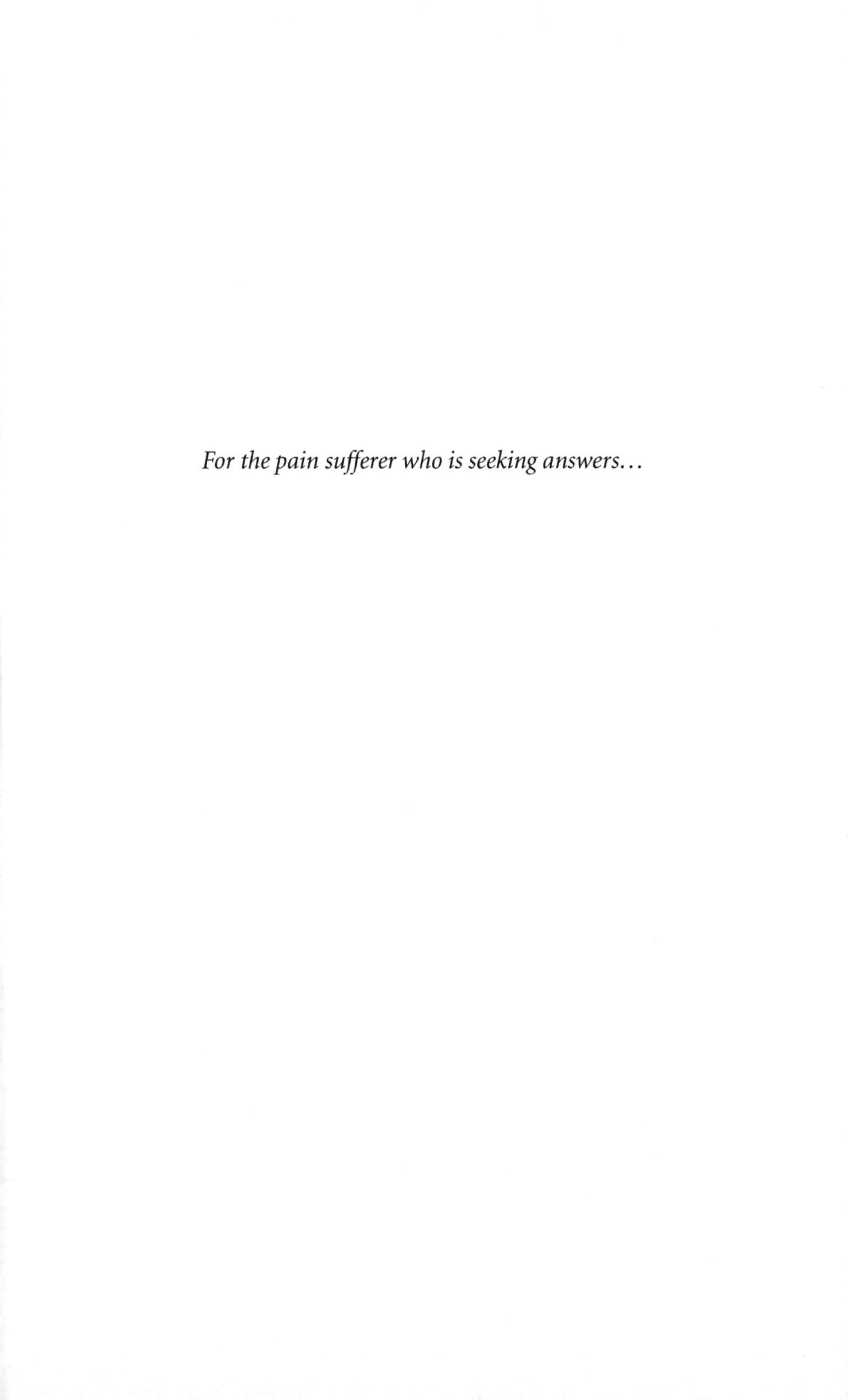

For the pain sufferer who is seeking answers…

Table of Contents

Foreword

She was tired, and not the normal end-of-the-workday kind of tired. It was a thoroughly exhausted deep in her bones kind of tired. A tired that drained the body of the energy to make the slightest move; a tired no amount of rest could cure. Knowing what I know now, that kind of tired is a sign of serious illness. Back then we didn't know what to do when my grandmother, Dorothy, started feeling this way.

Ever since my grandfather passed away, my Grandma Dorothy had been living with us. She was a feisty Norwegian with short white hair and an easy laugh whose love for baking was surpassed only by the love for her family and devotion to her faith. I remember coming home from school and waiting for me on the kitchen counter would be a batch of freshly baked cookies. I remember evenings when she would talk about the joys and hardships she and my grandfather faced raising five kids on a farm in northern Minnesota. I remember mornings when I would hear her pray for each one of her kids, grandkids, and great-grandkids by name. Those were the good days. We grew close over those years, which would make what happened to her something that was so unfair and painful, yet changed my life forever.

When her tiredness turned into extreme weakness and stomach discomfort we brought her to the hospital where doctors began running diagnostic tests—that was on a Sunday. The following

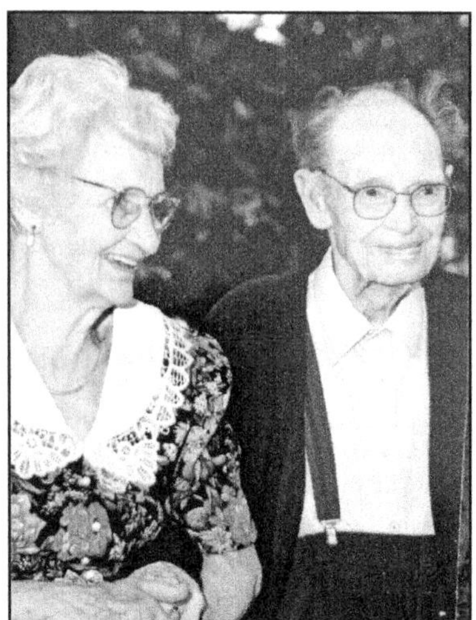
My grandfather, Norris Trontvet, and my grandmother, Dorothy.

Monday afternoon, while lying quietly on a hospital bed, it happened. The lining of her stomach burst, spilling acid into her abdominal cavity. Her screams of pain could be heard down the hallway. She writhed in so much agony and with such ferocity it took all the strength of two male nurses to hold down my tiny 87-year-old grandma.

Emergency surgery saved her life. The attending physician told us she had suffered a perforated ulcer caused, in all likelihood, by the medication she had been given. The next day, Tuesday, the tests results revealed the reason for her tiredness: bone cancer. She had survived the ulcer, but the cancer took her eleven days later.

I was twenty years old when that happened and well into my education for a career in healthcare. But when I heard of the pain my grandmother went through and the cause of it, I felt like I'd been hit with the full force and shock of a lightning bolt. There was a vivid illuminating moment of discovery that changed the course of my life. Right there and then I vowed to help people stay as far away from pain as much as possible and do it without prescribing medication with its potentially lethal side effects.

Half a decade later I graduated, one of the youngest in my class, with a Bachelor of Science in Human Biology and a Doctorate in Chiropractic. After I received my license allowing me to practice I thought I had finally arrived. I was going to be able to fulfill my mission.

How wrong I was.

Within months of taking over an existing clinic, it started to go under. I was losing patients and losing money. To a certain extent when a new doctor takes over another doctor's patients you always anticipate a "dip" but when the "dip" turned into a seemingly bottomless pit, I knew I was in trouble. The knowledge and skills I had acquired were "good enough," but apparently, no one wants to go to a doctor who's "good enough." And my staff must have felt the ship sinking because it didn't take long for them to quit.

So, there I was, patients disappearing, no support staff, and my income in jeopardy with student loans coming due. Worst of all, I couldn't shake the feeling that I had failed. I had gotten so close to fulfilling my vow of helping people regain their health and be pain-free, but had fallen embarrassingly short. The lowest point was the morning when I woke up late—twenty minutes before my first patient—and I couldn't get out of bed. I had a horrible gnawing feeling in my gut that I had made the wrong decision in becoming a chiropractor. What was I going to do?

Then the phone rang. It was my mentor, calling to see how I was doing. I told him everything. After a moment of silence (a pause that seemed like eternity to me) he said, "Ben, you're going to get beat up. That's life. The world is set up to make you fail, but you have a choice. You can stay in bed or you can believe that you were put on this Earth for a purpose and a mission. I've been through some hell in my life and I can tell you from experience that you've been given a spirit of power and if you do decide to use it, it will give you the strength to get up, pursue your goals, and live out your purpose to the best of your ability. And then, at the end of the day, you can go to sleep listening to the applause in Heaven, being grateful for what you accomplished that day, and hope for the chance to wake up tomorrow and do it all again."

I sat up in bed listening intently as he continued, "You do not attract into your life what you want. You only attract who you are. Now get to work."

That was another lightning bolt moment. In that moment, I decided I was going to be the best doctor I could be. (And in case you're wondering, yes, I was very late to that patient's appointment.)

I knew there were health professionals providing superior care and getting amazing results so I vowed to find them, study their methods, and bring that skill to my clinic and my community. I bought textbooks, old and new, from my profession and other professions. I got up at 3:45 a.m. to study them. I listened to CDs, podcasts, audio books—anything and everything I could get my hands on that would help me deliver a higher standard of care. All of this to the dismay of my wife—a light sleeper and not a morning person. I went further afield. I also traveled throughout the country listening to leaders in the world of spinal health, recovery, and pain relief.

While attending a workshop in Canada led by Dr. James Chestnut, one of the top minds in spinal health, I realized the answer to eliminating back and neck problems was not just chiropractic but rather in comprehensive physical care—therapeutic exercises tailored to the individual person and their lifestyle, advanced hands-on muscle therapy that targeted specific tissues, and nutrition. As a result I became a better doctor and my clinic started to grow.

But I knew I was still missing something. I didn't find it until I read Dr. Kelly Starrett's book "Becoming a Supple Leopard." Until then I had focused on the most effective treatment for back and neck pain, but I hadn't figured out how to prevent it. That groundbreaking book started me on a track of further study that made me realize we must use our backs and necks better along with complete physical care to really live a pain-free life.

Once this piece fell into place and I had the right team, my clinic grew to be the largest chiropractic clinic in the county (admittedly it is a smaller county in Minnesota, but nevertheless something I could be proud of). Then, in 2015, out of a group of over four hundred clinics across the nation, I was recognized as the Associate Doctor of the Year, and most recently, in 2016, my clinic was awarded the Patient's Choice Award.

Those awards were cool and I was happy to get the recognition, but that wasn't what mattered most to me. What mattered most was 1) seeing people get out of pain without drugs and surgery, and 2) being able to walk past the pictures of Grandma Dorothy, my head held high, knowing that I'm living my purpose, upholding my vow, and providing my community with the absolute best protocols to eliminate back and neck pain.

This book is the most recent manifestation of that journey.

—Dr. Ben Grams, D.C.

About the Author

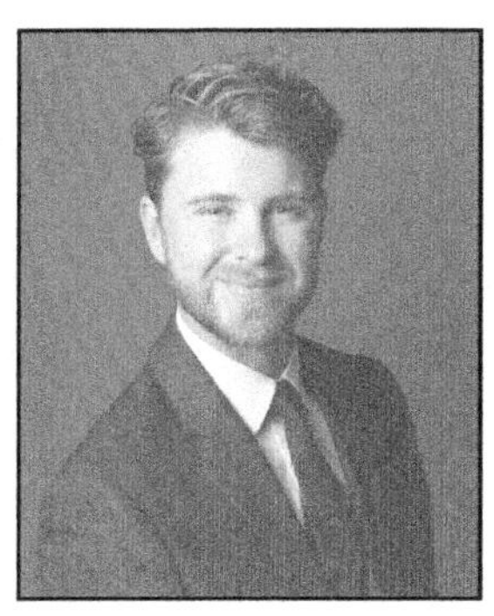

Ben Grams, DC, is an award-winning chiropractic physician and frequent event speaker. He is a champion of evidence-based and patient-centered healthcare with a long track record of helping people eliminate pain and regain their health by integrating the best of the holistic and medical worlds. His clinic, HealthSource Chiropractic and Progressive Rehab, is located in Little Falls, Minnesota, where he has practiced since 2011.

Dr. Grams' ultimate mission is to better the world by helping individuals transform their health and improve their quality of life. He believes that the only way to change a person's health is to change the way they think about health.

Dr. Grams' commitment to this mission is surpassed only by his discipleship to Christ Jesus and love for his family as a devoted husband, and a loving son, brother, and uncle.

Follow Dr. Grams on Facebook, Twitter, and YouTube. For more information, contact drbengrams@gmail.com.

Introduction

The more I came to know about the pain industry, the less I wanted to know.

I didn't *want* to realize how powerful and profitable pharmaceutical companies have become—or how strongly they influence our healthcare system. I didn't *want* to see the extremes of chiropractic—on one side, philosophical arrogance, and on the other, weak-kneed ignorance—and how they've stretched thin the profession. And, I certainly I didn't *want* to feel the separation of the decades-wide chasm that exists between the medical community and nearly every other form of healing.

I didn't *want* to know all this because, day in and day out, I was looking into the eyes of people in pain who the healthcare system had failed. I saw the hurt, the limitations, and the lack of a good life they were being forced to suffer through. It bothered me then, almost as much as it bothers me now.

And as time went on and more patients came through my door, I became increasingly aware of the problem at hand: 1) the standard approach to back and neck pain fails to address the *cause* of that pain, and 2) little-to-no action is taken to *prevent* pain. The frustrating bit is that the solution is so simple, but, once again, it seems the pain industry's "powers that be" have become too focused on their bottom line to see it, too lost in their legalism to find a way out, or are simply too stubborn to change.

This brings me to why I wrote this book. I want to help as many people as I can to get rid of pain, and stop it from ever coming back (or better yet, prevent it from occurring in the first place.) You, the reader, are giving me the chance to do that, and for that I am grateful.

Here's what to expect: this book reveals the shocking truth behind the "pain industry," and the simple steps you can take to *banish pain from your life.* Written to be informative, easy-to-read and yet, scientifically based, *The Solution to Back and Neck Pain That No One is Telling You About* will show you how to:

- Harness the powerful science behind the central nervous system to quickly propel yourself out of pain.
- Avoid making the costly and painful mistake of going to the wrong doctor or undergoing the wrong treatment.
- Spot a clever (and empty) sales pitch from a mile away—one selling a "magic bullet" for pain—saving you time, money, and frustration.
- Rid your life of empty diagnoses like "pain is normal at your age," and "there's nothing you can do about it."
- Figure out what you're doing (that you shouldn't) that got you in so much pain in the first place. This is an absolutely crucial skill needed to eliminate pain.
- Live everyday as pain free as possible through utilizing a handful of daily, commonsense habits.

Lastly, *The Solution to Back and Neck Pain That No One is Telling You About* delivers a new and proven method for going from dysfunction to function, from hurting to healing, from pain-full-ness to pain-*free*-ness in a way that is safer and cheaper than pills, injections, and surgeries. It is bold and educational, and its contents will be shocking and disturbing for many readers, but it offers a solution for all back and neck pain sufferers.

SECTION 1

All About Pain

One of the most tragic events of our time is that we know more about the pains and sufferings of the world and yet are less and less able to respond to them.—Henri Nouwen

NOT IF I HAVE SOMETHING TO SAY ABOUT IT!

-DR. BEN GRAMS

Chapter 1

Pain: It Hurts More Than You Might Think

"Your new patient is waiting in the exam room," my assistant announced. "And Dr. Grams, his wife wanted me to tell you that he's been dealing with some *really bad* lower back pain."

"Okay. Thanks for the heads up," As I opened his file to study its contents, I noticed out of the corner of my eye that she was lingering in the doorway. "Is there something else, Christy?"

"She also wanted me to warn you...he *really* doesn't want to be here."

"Great," I muttered as I walked into the room where he waited. "You must be Henry. I'm Dr. Ben Grams." I tried not to grimace as he practically squeezed all of my metacarpal bones together when we shook hands. "Welcome to the clinic, and thank you for coming."

His file showed he was an active-duty serviceman, stationed at a nearby military camp, and the variety of patches on his combat fatigues meant he had probably seen his share of combat. His uniform, although somewhat loose, couldn't hide his powerful physique—a thick neck, broad shoulders, and a chest that looked like he did more pushups in one day than I could manage in a year. As I sat across from him, he crossed his enormous arms over his chest and glared at me, his lips set in a firm line.

I held my clipboard and readied myself for what looked like a hard question-answer session. "Can you show me where you're feeling the pain?"

Leaning forward, he briefly pointed to his lower back, "Here."

"What does it feel li—?"

"It hurts," he grunted before I could finish asking the question.

I made a note in his file. "When did it start?"

"A long time ago."

"How did it come on?"

"Not sure," he answered, rolling his eyes.

"How often does it bother you?"

"All the time."

I felt like he really wanted to add "idiot" to the end of that last answer, but I ignored his cold glower and pressed on.

"Does the pain radiate anywhere?"

"No."

"Have you found anything that helps relieve the pain?"

"No."

"How about anything that makes it worse?" *Or anything else to say, other than no?*

"No."

Something wasn't adding up. Henry didn't seem like the type of man who would waste his time sitting in a doctor's office for no reason. I wanted to know why he was here, so I pressed a little harder.

I looked up from my notes. "How is your pain interfering with your life?"

No response.

"Henry?"

Dropping his head and letting out a deep sigh, he uncrossed his arms. "Normal things, doc."

As an expert in the human frame, I know there's truth behind the saying that body language expresses more than words, and that the uncrossing of the arms meant he was ready to open up more. This was my chance. So I stuck my pen behind my ear and asked, "Like what? Give me an example."

"Like tying my shoes or mowing the lawn." Henry shifted in his seat. "I can't even sit for more than five minutes before the pain gets worse, for crying out loud." He inhaled as if he was going to continue speaking, but nothing followed.

He ran his fingers through his buzz-cut hair. As he did, something changed in the very air of that room. It was as though he was battening down—hiding, protecting what lay beneath. After a moment, I asked, "What else?"

He shrugged, eyes darting to the door as though he longed to escape. "I dunno. What do you mean?"

"How else would you say that your pain has stopped you from doing what you want to do, or being what you want to be? In your home life, your work—anything." I pulled the pen from behind my ear, preparing to note any information that could follow. But information didn't follow. Only more silence, punctuated by worry in the back of my mind that I'd offended him somehow. Maybe he thought I was prying into his personal life or perhaps implying he was inadequate in some way.

I looked up, anxiety constricting my throat. But Henry wasn't red in the face, ready to go to blows with the chiropractor he never wanted to visit in the first place. Instead, his brow was scrunched, and deep lines creased his downcast face.

Over the years, I would come to learn that my patients didn't always realize how deeply their own wounds ran. In that moment, however, I didn't realize it either. So I sat there, uncomfortably waiting for him to speak.

He let out another sigh, "I guess..." Henry's eyes now studied his calloused hands as they folded together and his thumbs began a rhythmic twiddling. "Then there are my two boys." His voice cracked as he spoke. His eyes welled up with tears—tears he fought to blink away and hide at all costs. I wanted to lean forward and place a comforting hand on his shoulder; to let him know there was no shame in what he felt. Before I could, he continued, "I feel like... like...I'm failing as a father. I can't play or wrestle with them. I have to keep telling them, 'Daddy can't do that right now.' And what they don't know is that, with the way that my back has been going over the past few years, I probably won't be able to do it...ever."

I had to blink away a few tears myself when he revealed that.

Clearing his throat and regaining his military-like composure, he said, "Sorry. It's that they're the best thing that has ever happened to me, and I feel like I'm missing out on their lives. I don't want that." Then he chuckled at himself and shook his head. "Guess that wife of mine was right, my back really *is* that bad."

I had been studying the human body for nearly a decade, with a keen interest on pain for much of that time. But in that moment, I realized that while pain physically hurts, it's what pain does to us—what it *steals from us*—that makes it hurt the most.

I wish I could say that Henry's story is unique, but it's not. Pain has become something of a national preoccupation. You'll find it's a frequent topic of conversation with family and friends. It seems like no matter where you go, pain is there—mostly because the number of those suffering with it is spiraling out of control. More people are diagnosed with back and neck pain than heart disease, diabetes, and cancer, making it one of the top reasons people seek medical attention.[1,2] Unfortunately, the attention they receive isn't doing the trick. More medications are prescribed, injections administered, and surgeries performed than ever before, yet the number of pain sufferers keeps rising.

It's obvious that we're missing something.

Pain robs us of sleep, depletes bank accounts, ruins relationships, and smothers intimacy. I've seen first-hand the devastation pain causes in people's lives. Some are completely blindsided by it, while others refuse to heed warning signs, repeatedly telling themselves "it's not that bad" until it *gets* that bad.

Here are some examples:

- ✓ I've talked to a grief-stricken grandmother who couldn't hold her newborn granddaughter because of shoulder pain.
- ✓ I've watched a teenager drop her head in shame while she admits her grades are slipping because her daily headaches steal her focus.
- ✓ I've seen preventable sports injuries cause months of training go down the drain moments before a big event.
- ✓ I've listened to a mother describe how guilty she feels for missing out on tender moments with her children.
- ✓ I've talked to people who simply want to be able to get out of bed, stand and talk to a friend, take a car trip, ride a bike, go for a walk, or simply sit and rest without pain.

These people want to live life, but pain has stopped them.

I've listened to their stories of attempts to find a solution, followed by failure. They go from one doctor to another, each one telling them something different, each one trying something different, but each one getting the same result: brief relief followed by persistent pain.

My goal in this book is to change that.

If you are in pain, hear this clearly: You do not have to be in misery, forced to undergo dangerous or ineffective treatments, waiting for some type of medicinal miracle to save you. I believe you should be able to live your life with little-to-no pain. I believe that you should be able to do what you want without pain stopping you. Furthermore, I believe the potential for you to be pain-free is already within you and simply needs to be released.

As you read this book, you may often find yourself asking, "How come I didn't know about this before?" You will also gain insights that will change your views on pain forever. And by the time you reach the final page of this book, you will understand exactly what you need to do to be pain-free.

Curious? Good. The journey to becoming pain-free starts now.

Chapter 2

The First Step to Becoming Pain-Free

A journey of a thousand miles begins with a single step.
—Chinese Proverb

When an outside force is causing your pain, getting rid of it is usually accomplished in one step. Your finger is jammed in a door? Open it. You're touching a hot iron? Stop touching it. Your feet hurt because your shoes don't fit? Take them off.

But when there's an inside force causing your pain—like when there's something wrong with the body itself—eliminating pain can't be accomplished in one fell swoop.

The dilemma we face is that when we're in pain, our number one priority is getting out of it. Not tomorrow. Not next week. But right now. This urgency is our enemy if the goal is to genuinely rid ourselves of back and neck pain, especially if that pain is chronic. Don't get me wrong. I'm all for eliminating pain quickly and easily, but the fact remains that if we try to eliminate pain without taking the proper steps, we're going to be both frustrated and *still in pain.*

The Steps to Becoming Pain-Free:

- ✓ Expose the Myths
- ✓ Learn the Basics
- ✓ Understand the Problem
- ✓ Discover The Solution
- ✓ Take Action

Each component is a step in the right direction to bringing you closer to a world in which pain is greatly diminished—maybe even banished. I am going to be your guide, but in order to get to your desired destination, *you* have to take the first step.

Are you ready?

Turn the page.

SECTION 2

Pain Myths: Exposing Lies and Revealing the Truth

The truth is like a lion. You don't have to defend it. Let it loose. It will defend itself.—St. Augustine

Chapter 3

MYTH 1: Pain Medication—"Take This, It Will Help You"

Drugs never cure disease. They merely hush the voice of nature's protest and pull down the danger signals she erects along the pathway of transgression. Any poison taken into the system has to be reckoned with later on even though it palliates present symptoms. Pain may disappear but the patient is left in a worse condition, though unconscious of it at the time. —Daniel Kraus, M.D.

Sometimes Healing Hurts

"Sticks and stones may break my bones, but words will never hurt me." I can't help but think how off-the-mark this phrase really is. The words we use do matter. Words carry meaning and wield incredible power.

Big drug companies are well aware of this. They know that the more they say a drug can do, the more money that drug will make. In fact, they've been working this angle for so long that they've figured out it takes only two words.

These two words have become their very own "Old Faithful" because they turn people like you into lifelong, gushing geysers of cash. These two words are the reason why after an injury, coaches, trainers, nurses, and doctors tell you to "take something for the pain." These two words are the reason why people who would prefer not to take anything for pain, go ahead and do so, telling themselves, "It's better safe than sorry." Oh, they *will be sorry.*

Sticks and stones may break your bones, yes, but these two words will hurt you and will leave you suffering from more pain than ever before. What are those two words? *Help you.* They say pain medication will ***help you***. It'll *help you* feel better. It'll *help you* heal better. It'll *help you* recover faster. And it can also *help you* prevent pain and injury.

It's a bunch of baloney, folks, and here's the evidence.

Order in the Court

Most people understand that pain medications such as aspirin, Aleve, Advil, and ibuprofen are designed to stop inflammation. The name of their drug class is a giveaway: non-steroidal *anti-inflammatory* drugs (NSAIDs). What very few realize is that by doing so, they also stop one of your most important allies in the fight against pain.

Exhibit A: Fibroblasts

Fibroblasts are specialized cells that help heal soft-tissue injuries. Here's how they work: When a ligament or tendon gets injured—whether it be a minor strain or a major tear—chemicals are released, causing inflammation. These chemicals seal off the injury site from foreign invaders, increase blood flow, and activate fibroblasts. When this happens, these cells go to work laying down new tissue to replace what has been damaged. Once their job is finished, the injury is repaired, and the ligament or tendon works as good as ever.

How well do NSAIDs *help* fibroblasts?

A 1995 study from the *American Journal of Sports Medicine* proved that an NSAID can stop a fibroblast dead in its tracks. After injury, patients treated with an NSAID showed no signs that fibroblasts were repairing damage. You see, by stopping inflammation, NSAIDs actually stopped the healing process.[1]

And it doesn't end there.

This isn't a problem only for ligaments and tendons, but also for muscles and cartilage. NSAIDs have been shown to interfere with the healing of soft tissue at every possible turn. So much so that in 2013, the *Open Rehabilitation Journal* published a study (which reviewed 203 other studies) concluding that NSAIDs should simply not be used for acute or chronic soft tissue injuries.[2]

For decades, mounds of evidence have piled up proving that pain meds hinder rather than help the healing process. Yet they are still a centerpiece in the standard medical treatment for injury and pain. Drug giants still advertise them. Doctors still recommend and prescribe them. And we all still have bottles and bottles of them in the medicine cabinet. This is bad for you and your health, but good for drug companies and their pocketbooks.

Exhibit B: Nociceptors (no-see-sep-tors)

A nociceptor is a special type of nerve that detects damage. All nerves conduct electrical signals to the brain. When the brain receives a signal from a nociceptor, it realizes that the body has been injured. To stop the injury from worsening, the brain converts a nociceptor's "damage" signal into pain. Pain, then, forces you to take action to get out of harm's way. For example:

- You stub your toe, nociceptors fire, you feel pain, and you make sure you avoid that corner next time.
- You roll your ankle, nociceptors fire, you feel pain, and you ease up on that ankle.
- You give yourself a paper cut, nociceptors fire, you feel pain, and you don't do it again.

To be clear, nociceptors do not conduct pain signals—they conduct damage signals. It's your brain that decides whether or not these signals turn into pain. This difference is important because it's why pain medications like Vicodin, hydrocodone, or acetaminophen (found in Tylenol) can actually make you feel more pain, not less.

Let me explain.

These medications block your brain from interpreting a nociceptor's signal as pain, which is why you feel better after taking them. Their downfall is that they don't turn off nociceptors. Those nerves keep firing, and eventually they get used so much they become "sensitized," meaning that it becomes ridiculously easy for them to fire more signals. How much easier? In 1997, the *Journal on Manipulative and Physiologic Therapeutics* discovered that "sensitization" increased firing "100-fold" making nociceptors capable of interpreting light touch and normal, day-to-day movement as damage—which "can lead to increased pain, muscle spasm, and reduced blood flow." [3]

In other words, the longer the problem causing the pain is covered up, the worse the problem gets, and the longer you'll be in pain—and eventually things that shouldn't hurt, will. To the point that if you ever try to get off the meds, guess what you're left with?

More pain. Or if your body builds a tolerance to the meds (which it always does), guess what you're left with? That's right, more pain.

That doesn't sound like the kind of *help* you need.

The Verdict

At best, pain medications provide temporary relief. At worst they leave you drugged, weakened, and in more pain. That's why those two words, "help you," are so dangerous. Pain meds *do not* help you heal, and anyone who tells you otherwise either doesn't know or doesn't care. Next time you hear "take something for the pain, it will help you," think twice and consider if that's the kind of help you really need.

Summary

- **MYTH:** Take something for the pain; it will *help you.* Those last two words are the big drug companies' ploy to get you to buy more. This is a dangerous myth because it has the ability to undermine your body's healing process. Be careful.
- **Fibroblasts** are special cells that repair you after you're injured. NSAIDs simply get in their way.
- **Sensitization** is a disease process where your **nociceptors**—nerves that detect damage—become high strung. If this sets in, you're in for a world of hurt.
- **TRUTH:** Pain meds do not help you heal. At best, they help you feel better temporarily. Be sure not to confuse the two.*

* This chapter, as well as the ones that follow, are not intended as a substitute for the medical advice of physicians. The reader should consult a physician in matters relating to his/her health and before making any changes to prescribed medications or procedures.

Chapter 4

Myth 2: Pain Medication—"Your Pain Will Simply Disappear"

Why is it that you're forced to simply EXPECT a laundry list of side effects if you start a new pain medication? Why is it that millions of people every day are watching commercials where the list of side effects is longer than the commercial itself...yet STILL spend their hard-earned money on those products? And why is it that millions of people all around the world are still willing to ACCEPT these dreadful, mind-fogging, life-shortening side effects even though there is a safer alternative available?—Jesse Cannone, Back Pain Specialist, Co-Founder of the Healthy Back Institute

A Spoonful of Money Makes the Medicine Go Down

Whenever you watch TV, it's there. Browse the internet, it's there, too. Skim through a magazine, read a newspaper, or listen to the radio, and you run into it. In fact, unless you've been hiding under a rock for the past few years, you've encountered a deadly, bold-faced lie hundreds of times.

Before I tell you what it is, let me tell you who's behind it.

Those pulling the strings are the deep-pocketed, profit-driven drug companies. One of their "oldest tricks in the book" is using their cold hard cash to keep their claws buried deep in everything that we watch, read, and hear. We're talking $19 billion a year spent on advertising, folks.[4] That's $1.58 billion a month…$365 million a week…$52 million per day…$2.17 million per hour…$36,149 per minute! All this is to make sure what you hear about their drugs is exactly what they want you to hear.

What is more disconcerting is the fact that a 2012 study, published in the prestigious *British Medical Journal*, revealed that these gigantic medication corporations are spending a lot more on advertising than they spend on basic research. Not double, triple, or quadruple. They spend nineteen times[5] more money convincing you to buy their meds than they do trying to improve them. Doesn't that seem wrong to you? Shouldn't this be the other way around?

It seems these drug companies view pain sufferers as a cash crop ripe for the picking. One of their harvesting methods is to flood the media with a myth so sinister that the only thing more gut-wrenching is the sheer number of people who have been blindsided by it. Here is the lie: "If you're in pain and you take a pill, the pain *simply* disappears." Good grief! Not true. Sure, pain pills can provide temporary relief, but they only mask the problem. The little known truth behind this myth is that by depending on these pills the only thing that "simply disappears" is your health!

A Bitter Pill to Swallow

"Big Pharma" has worked hard to make sure we recognize their products and they work even harder sweeping the dangerous and downright deadly side effects of these pills under the rug. Well, it's time *we* pull that rug out from under *them* and expose the truth.

> **Acetaminophen** (example: Tylenol and Excedrin): It's the deadliest over-the-counter pain reliever on the market[6], and the nation's leading cause of acute liver failure[7]. Federal data shows that every year this drug is responsible for sending as many as 78,000 Americans to the emergency room due to overdose[8]. This is partly because liver damage can occur from taking a smaller amount than you might think. According to the FDA, taken over several days, as little as 25 percent above the maximum daily dose of 4 grams (or just two additional extra strength pills a day) has been reported to cause liver damage.[9]
>
> **Ibuprofen, naproxen, aspirin** (example: Advil, Motrin, and Aleve): According to the *New England Journal of Medicine*, every year these drugs—non-steroidal anti-inflammatory drugs (NSAIDs)—cause at least 16,500 Americans to bleed to death, making them the 15th most common cause of death in the U.S.[10]

All of these over-the-counter pills are like traitorous double agents. On one hand, they're on your side providing temporary relief, but their true mission is to *simply* sabotage your health. Here an example of what I mean. If you take a thousand acetaminophen pills in your lifetime (less than two per month), you double your risk of your kidneys shutting down permanently.[11] And here's another one: In 2009, a study in the journal *Neurology* showed that those who took the most NSAIDs increased their risk of Alzheimer's by 66 percent.[12]

Of course, the drug giants have made darn sure these meds are never more than a hop, skip, and a jump away. But what about the pain meds that you can't pick up at your neighborhood convenience store? What about the ones that require a prescription?

Prescription drugs are obviously harder to obtain because you need your doctor to prescribe them—and you can't simply waltz into a drugstore, grab them off the shelf, and pop them to your heart's content. Nevertheless, in spite of that level of scrutiny and control, the amount of prescription medication consumed by Americans is mind-boggling. *Over a ten-year period* (1999–2010) *the number of prescription painkillers sold in doctors' offices and pharmacies quadrupled.* The Centers for Disease Control and Prevention (CDC) says that in the year 2010 alone, "Enough prescription pain killers were prescribed to medicate every American adult around-the-clock for a month."[13] Take a moment and let that soak in.

And while the potency of prescription medications makes them more effective at relieving pain, they also come with a smaller margin for error. Meaning, fewer pills can cause more damage. Which is the reason why a prescription is needed to obtain them in the first place. The prescription gives the doctor control over the dosage and therefore lessens the risks.

Simple, right?

But what if the doctors are misled? What if they aren't told the whole truth behind the medication they're prescribing? What havoc does the potency of these pain relievers wreak then? Take a deep breath because we're about to dive into two examples where that's exactly what happened:

> **Vioxx:** Distributed worldwide, this painkiller was considered to be a "blockbuster" because it averaged over a billion dollars in sales annually[14,15]—that's a lot of pills being sold. A short while after being on the market a major problem was found:

taking it skyrocketed the chances of heart attack or stroke by up to 500 percent![16] Did Merck, the developer, warn doctors of the risk and immediately pull it off the market? Nope. Not a chance. Because of a cat-and-mouse game so complex that entire books have been written about it, five years passed before it was finally taken off the market. By then, it was too late. The damage had already been done: it had contributed to between 88,000-140,000 heart attacks, about half of them fatal.[17] Blockbuster? More like executioner.

Celebrex: This drug was found to triple the risk of heart attack or stroke for those taking it.[18] But that's just the tip of the iceberg. Celebrex claimed to be easier on the stomach than more established drugs—a considerable selling point to doctors and patients alike. It even had a six-month study to prove it. Too bad it was all a hoax. You see, the actual study was for an entire year, but the researchers simply failed to mention the second half of that study which happen to prove that it wasn't better at protecting the stomach whatsoever. Why the smoke and mirrors? Perhaps it has something to do with Celebrex racking up more than $2.4 billion in sales.[19]

I hope you're starting to see that "take a pill and the pain will *simply* disappear" is as far from the truth as north is from south and that depending on pain meds to get through your day may be more beneficial for Big Pharma's pocket book than your health.

A side note: It's undeniable that both Vioxx and Celebrex relieved pain, but they did so while hurting a lot of people. In Part 5 of this book, I'm going to unveil a method to eliminate back and neck pain that is without *any* of the dangerous side effects and smoke-and-mirrors you've read about so far. Although you have a bit of reading to get through before you're there, while we're here now, let me whet your appetite by giving you a glimpse of the effectiveness of this method: a 2003 study published in the research journal *Spine* showed that just one component of this approach was 500 percent more effective at relieving chronic back and neck pain than either Vioxx or Celebrex.[20] Pretty exciting, huh?

The last type of prescription medication we'll address is one we've all know there's a problem with, but what you might not be aware of is how bad the problem has become.

> **Opioids** (for example: Vicodin, Oxycodone, Oxymorphone, Demerol, Percocet, Methadone, Hydrocodone, and Norco): If there were a "weapon of mass destruction" in the pain medication world, this would be it. How bad are these drugs? Dr. Gary Franklin, neurologist and medical director for Washington State Department of Labor & Industries, said, "We've seen more than 100,000 deaths between 1999 and 2010, almost twice as many as U.S. casualties in the Vietnam War. In addition, we have millions of people who have become dependent or addicted, who will never be off opioids, and who will never be helped by these drugs."
>
> And currently they're causing 15,000 deaths per year.[21] Their side effects are no walk in the park either ranging from drowsiness and dizziness to confusion, severe constipation, ruptured bowels, depression, coma, suffocation, and more pain.[22]

Let's take a quick time out and clear up one thing. I'm *not* saying that pain-suppressing drugs have *no* place in healthcare. When used at the right time and for the right reasons, pain medications are good. On the other hand, if we believe something as foolhardy as "If I'm in pain I can take a pill and it will *simply* disappear" chances are we will use pain meds at the wrong time and for the wrong reasons which can result in very serious problems. I think we all can agree on that. Dr. Virgil V. Strang, Dean of Philosophy and Director of Professional Ethics, Palmer College of Chiropractic, put it perfectly into perspective when he said, "It is one thing to offer pain suppressing drugs to a dying 85-year-old; it is quite different to administer pain killers to a 20-year-old who has fallen on his buttocks."

Certainly, there are times when taking something to help with the pain is absolutely necessary and there are other times when it's not. Knowing that difference and being aware of the risks involved is an important step toward getting your back and neck healthy and pain-free.

And the issues mentioned in this chapter are just the tip of the iceberg—not good news for pain sufferers.

You'll discover more by continuing on to next chapter.

Summary

- **MYTH:** "Take something for the pain, and it'll *simply* disappear." Drug companies have repeated this line for decades for one reason: to get you to buy their product so that they can make money. Don't fall for it. It's a lie. Pain medication may help you feel better, but it does so while leaving the cause of your pain unaddressed. It's a short-term fix, not a long-term solution.
- **TRUTH:** All pain medications have side effects. Some are worse than others, and all are worse than what Big Pharma wants us to believe. The way to get back and neck pain to

disappear is not found in a pill that overrides the body. It will, however, be found in a proven method that *works* with the body. It's as *simple* as that.

Chapter 5

Myth 3: "The Doctor Only Has My Best Interests in Mind"

Twisted together like the snake and the staff, doctors and drug companies have become entangled in a web of interactions as controversial as they are widespread.
—Arnold Relman, M.D., Harvard medical professor

When we go to the doctor, we assume they want only what's best for us—which is certainly true. The vast majority of doctors become doctors because they want to heal sick people. That much is obvious. What isn't as obvious, in fact what been hidden from public view, are the tactics big drug companies use to influence what's on the minds of our doctors when they see us.

Whatever amount of time, energy, and money Big Pharma spends on convincing me and you to buy their specific brands, that pales in comparison to the resources they devote to sway our doctors. Why? They know that doctors are the gatekeeper to our pocketbook because only they have the power to prescribe medication. So let's pull back the curtain and expose the truth behind this next myth.

Talk to Your Doctor

1) **Early bird gets the worm.** Drug companies know that getting in with doctors when they're younger is key to persuading those doctors to continue to prescribe their brand when they're older. That's why you find Big Pharma's presence at nearly every medical school across the country where students are provided with free pizza, pasta, pens, and all manner of perks. This may seem like no big deal, but that's exactly what they want you to believe. In 2004 the *New England Journal of Medicine* published an eye-opening article by a group of investigators who said that, "even small gifts create a sense of indebtedness, which can lead to inappropriate prescribing." [23] The old saying is true: there is no such thing as a free lunch.

2) **Train of Thought.** Not even the teachers and researchers can escape the reach of the drug giants' grasp. Like an infection, Big Pharma's influence has spread to the highest levels of research, making it nearly impossible to find a senior medical researcher who isn't in bed with them.[24] This is a problem because it's through research that doctors know what the best course of action is for you. Harvard professor Arnold Relman, a noted critic of the cozy relationship between medical practitioners and the drug industry, pulls no punches: "The medical profession is being bought by the pharmaceutical industry, not only in terms of the practice of medicine, but

also in terms of teaching and research." And later saying that, "Academic institutions of this country are allowing themselves to be paid agents of the pharmaceutical industry. I think it's disgraceful." [24] [†]

3) **Repetition. Repetition. Repetition.** Every day in the U.S. about 100,000 sales representatives visit doctors—ranging from family doctors to those in the ER.[25] Targeting doctors is considered so critical to the drug industry that they shell out at least $21,000 per doctor per year bombarding them with marketing material designed to persuade them to prescribe you their latest product.[26] This is the pharmaceutical companies' favorite marketing tool for one reason: it is unnervingly effective. You'll find out how good the return on their investment is in a moment. These tactics, though, have been going on for so long that one frustrated researcher said that "these aggressive, over-the-top marketing practices 'are virtual fixtures in medical practice.'" [23]

And that's not the scary part.

4) **The scary part is this:** while most doctors accept this is going on, most reject the possibility that it actually affects them. Yet another researcher, had this to say: "My criticism is of the naiveté of doctors and/or their unwillingness to accept overwhelming evidence that the techniques used by the industry to increase prescribing their products actually work." [27]

How well their tactics work is a lot more hair-raising.

Brace yourself.

[†] If you want to learn more about this or maybe you don't believe me, I suggest reading the research article that is referenced in this paragraph. It's absolutely startling.

The Return on Investment (ROI)

Since the early 1990s, the number of prescriptions that Americans consume has nearly doubled.[28] In 2011 this came to roughly thirteen prescriptions for every man, woman, and child.[29] When you boil this down, it means that we are consuming 25 million pills… not per year…not per week…not per day…*but per hour.*[30]

That's a lot of medication. And for the ever-greedy drug companies, that's a lot of money. Since 1997, the amount Americans spend on prescription drugs has increased 392 percent.[24] And in 2015 the drug giants generated a whopping $309.5 billion.[31] If you were to have that amount of money in one hundred dollar bills stacked end-to-end, it would reach the moon's surface. And, you'd still have millions left over.

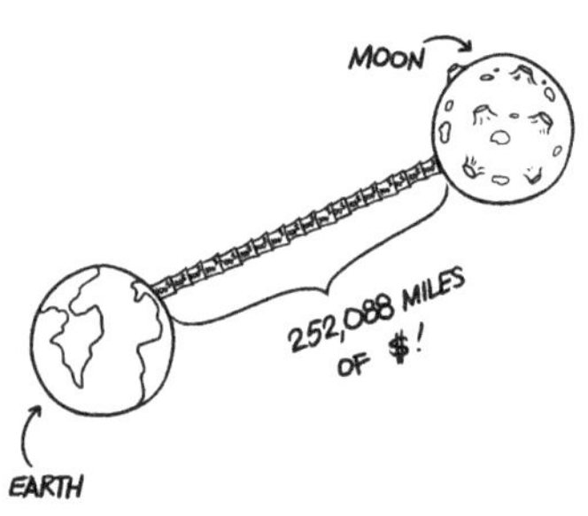

It's obvious that drug companies do not have your best interests in mind. As said earlier, their main interest is making money. But what about our doctors who are caught in the middle of all this?

The Truth

Let me be clear. *Doctors are caring and smart people who are where they are and do what they do because they want to help people like me and you.* Doctors *do* have your best interests in mind, but they're busy and overloaded with patients. Plus, there is an overwhelming onslaught of new research to absorb almost daily. And they can't learn *everything* in all their years at med school. So when you combine all of this with Big Pharma's influence in schools, hospitals, and clinics, it's impossible that your best interests are the *only* thing on your doctor's mind.

What do you do? I will show you exactly what to do to become pain-free throughout this book, but for right now, rest assured that being aware of this myth as you seek help with your pain is part of the solution.

Summary

- **MYTH:** *Doctors have only your best interests in mind.* Doctors are targeted early and often by the major drug corporations in a relentless attempt to persuade them to use the products that they sell.
- **TRUTH:** Doctors do have your best interests in mind, but it's not the *only thing on* their mind. So if you're in pain and you're headed to the doctor or any other healthcare professional's office, recognize that they're human and not without flaws.

Chapter 6

Myth 4: "Doctor Knows Best"

"Doctors are great—as long as you don't need them."
—Edward E. Rosenbaum, author "A Taste of My Own Medicine: When the Doctor Is the Patient"

If you're like most people, when there's a problem with your health, you call the doctor—and for good reason. Right? After all, it's well known that doctors invest years learning all about the human body and have by far the most experience. It's understandable, therefore, that as a group, they are regarded as the foremost authority on health. That's why since your childhood, it's been drummed into you to "follow your doctor's orders" and "do as the doctor says." The drug industry certainly recognizes their authority by ending every commercial with the same line: "Talk to your doctor to see if our drug is right for you."

And, in many, many circumstances it's absolutely true that "doctor knows best."

There is one instance where it is often not true, and that's when you're in pain. In her book, *A Nation in Pain,* Judy Foreman tells us that: "Pain is the main reason that patients go to doctors, but most doctors know almost nothing about it, much less how to treat it."

How can this be? How come the people who are the authority on the human body know alarmingly little about pain?

Back to School

It goes back to doctors' days at med school when they are taught less about pain than you'd expect (and hope). Let me be the first to acknowledge: Becoming a doctor is no small feat. Thousands of hours are spent in classrooms learning everything from chemical reactions to how to do CPR. On top of that, a would-be doctor spends untold hours studying outside of the classroom, not to mention the seemingly never-ending hoops they have to jump through: pop quizzes, reports, midterms, finals, and expensive board exams. Trust me, I've been there, and it's exhausting.

That's part of the reason why I was shocked when I read what the John Hopkins Pain Curriculum Development Team found and published in *The Journal of Pain* (2011) about the amount of time devoted to teaching medical students about pain, and how to treat it. Here's a direct quote: "A large number of U.S. medical schools are not reporting *any* teaching of pain." The emphasis is mine here because it's so hard to believe. Even in the "better" medical schools, the average time spent on pain education is only nine hours.[32] That's not nine hours a semester or nine hours a year—that's nine hours stretched over four years. You can't get good at playing the kazoo in nine hours, much less learn the ins and outs of pain relief.

Before I go any further, please don't feel I'm taking cheap shots at my brethren medical practitioners. Other healthcare specialties like chiropractic, physical therapy, massage therapy, and acupuncture have their own shortcomings when it comes to pain education. For example, a sizable sector in chiropractic considers pain a four-letter-word not to be repeated. "We don't treat pain. We only eliminate subluxations[‡]" is the mantra they shout. I've even heard practice management groups advise to not talk about pain because "once the pain is gone, the patient is gone." All the while, millions of Americans are having difficulty getting out of bed in the morning.

It's absolute madness!

Perhaps you'd like to know who gets closer to ninety hours of pain education during their training? Veterinarians.[33] This means that Fido has a better chance of getting rid of his back pain than you do.

In the Field

But what about doctors once they are in the trenches, seeing patients day in and day out? You can be excused for thinking that they will quickly compensate for the shortfalls in the education system and get up to speed. But you'll want to think again. Pouring more salt on the wound, a 2007 study published in the *American Journal of Medical Sciences,* which involved twelve medical research centers, revealed that, out of 500 doctors who were seeing patients, only one-third felt comfortable treating someone who had chronic pain.[34] This means that if you've been suffering from a pain for more than three months, chances are your doctor has to take a deep breath and gather his thoughts before walking into the examination room with you.

‡ Subluxation is a medical term used to describe a dysfunctional spinal joint that interferes with the nervous system.

Not good news for pain sufferers, and not breaking news to the healthcare industry.

In a major report, the Institute of Pain recognized that: "Most people are cared for by primary care physicians who likely received little initial training or experience in best practices for pain management." They continue, "Too many physicians harbor outmoded or unscientific attitudes toward pain and people with pain."[35]

Most doctors (and there are exceptions to the rule) are not your best choice when it comes to the treatment of pain.

Hammer and Nail

That being said, some doctors are specially trained to handle pain. When it comes to them, it's no longer a matter of "*Does* the doctor know how to get me out of pain?" but rather "*HOW does* the doctor know how to get me out of pain?" You need to know what to look for in a specialist doctor so you don't ruin your chances of ever becoming pain-free.

> ***"I suppose it is tempting, if the only tool you have is a hammer, everything looks like a nail."***
> ***—Dr. Abraham Maslow, psychologist***

When a doctor is trained in a certain way, she filters problems and conditions through that training. A surgeon, for example, has a surgical filter. When a person with neck or back pain goes to a surgeon, that doctor's job is to determine whether or not surgery is a good option. If you go to a physical therapist, it's the same thing. With their physical therapy filter, their job is to determine if physical therapy is a good option. This rule applies across all of healthcare, ranging from neurologists to nurses to naturopaths.

What's the problem here?

The problem, and it's a big one, is that because of this, healthcare professionals tend to make patients fit the treatment they offer, instead of ensuring that the treatment fits the patient. That's part of the reason why nearly 25 percent of all medical procedures and tests are considered unnecessary—which affects tens of thousands of people and costs millions of dollars.[36, 37] The bottom line: many things seem like "good" options, but only a few things are the "right" option.

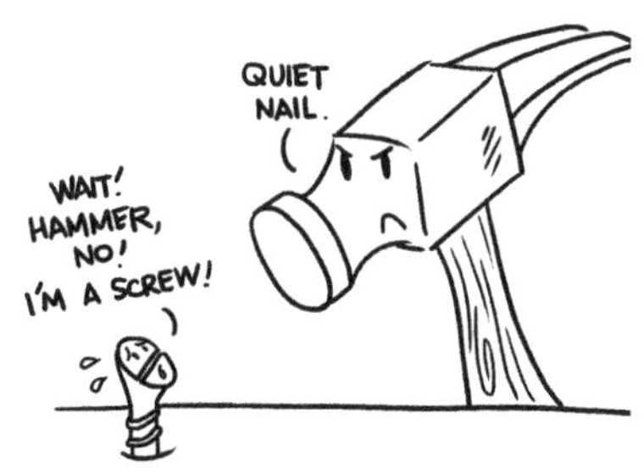

This is particularly true when it involves back and neck pain. Take the word of Gordon Waddell, an international authority on back and neck pain, when he says, "Much of the health care we give for back pain is inappropriate. Too often, the choice of treatment reflects the skills of the professional rather than the needs of the patient. To put it simply, what treatment you receive depends more on who you go to see than on what is wrong with your back."[38]

Pain sufferers, how do you know if the health professional you call for an appointment is going to give you the care you need? Keep reading. In Section 5: "Discover The Solution," I will tell you the exact kind of treatment proven to be the best, as well as the exact kind of specialist to seek in order to ensure that the treatment is designed specifically *for you*. Finding this person is worth immensely more than the cost of this book alone.

Stick with me here. We're making good time uncovering these pain myths and exposing the truth. If you've been suffering from back and neck pain, sooner or later, you'll reach a point where enough is enough. You're willing to try almost about anything, which sets you up perfectly for the next pain myth.

Let's bring to light Myth 5…

Summary

- **MYTH:** "The doctor knows best." Considering all of the education it takes to become a doctor, and taking into account that pain is one of the main reasons people seek medical attention, you would think that a doctor would know the best way to eliminate your pain. Unfortunately, for the most part, that isn't the case.
- **TRUTH:** A significant percentage of healthcare professionals receive an upsettingly small amount of education about pain, and this is compounded by the limitations that come with their specialty. It is crucial to find the right doctor or specialist who can provide the right treatment to become pain-free.

Chapter 7

MYTH 5: Invasive Procedures—"In Pain? Yeah, There's a Procedure for That"

Since when did we start asking "I wonder WHICH medication or procedure is right for me?" instead of asking the real question "I wonder IF medications or procedures are right for me?"

—Dr. Ben Grams

Watch Your Step

Millions have bought into the lie that if one medication doesn't relieve your pain, another one will. It may have to be stronger. You may need a doctor's prescription. It may cost you an arm and a leg—heck, you may have to insert, infuse, or inject that medication into your arm and your leg—but, by golly, it's going to work.

Pain sufferers aren't the only ones who have fallen for this lie; the whole pain industry, including most doctors, have too. We've come to think that the answer to back and neck pain is 1) better forms of medication delivered more specifically and/or 2) technology applied more directly. When ice, rest, pain pills, and muscle relaxants—the standard medical approach for back and neck pain—have failed (big surprise) the next step is onto a slippery slope: invasive procedures.

"Insanity: Doing the same thing over and over and expecting a different result" —Albert Einstein

Before I explain how all medications and invasive procedures—which is any treatment that requires the breaking of skin for direct entry into the body—are fundamentally flawed and will never, *ever* be able to get you pain-free I want to bust a myth behind a type of treatment that is performed on thousands of pain sufferers every day.

For nearly half a century, chemicals ranging from Botox (a toxin that paralyzes muscle) to lidocaine (what dentists use to numb your teeth) have been loaded into syringes and injected into the sorest spots of people's necks and backs, such as the:

- Epidural space: the area surrounding your spinal cord (the procedure is better known as an "epidural.")
- Facets: small joints that stabilize your spine.
- Trigger points: ultra-knotted parts of tight muscle.
- Nerve: the nerve that is transmitting the pain (the procedure is better known as a "nerve block.")

The whole idea is to inject numbing chemicals into the painful areas...and hope for the best. Please, don't fall victim to this myth. These procedures are not all they're cracked up to be.

First, they come with substantial side effects, including bleeding ulcers, bone death, osteoporosis, and infection. Second, millions have undergone these procedures only to have their hopes of pain-free living dashed.

Here's why:

- **You might as well be injected with salt water.** In 2009, a study headed by Richard Deyo, MD, professor and co-editor of the book *Evidence-Based Clinical Practice* found that corticosteroid injections (more commonly known as cortisone) were no more effective at relieving low back pain than "sham" injections that used only salt water.[39] A 2011 study published in the *British Medical Journal* showed the same.[40]
- **If you get relief, it's not going to last.** If injections succeed in actually numbing you, that relief, on average, lasts only eight to twelve weeks.[41] Why such a short time? Because the underlying problem causing the pain is still there, but you can't feel it. That's why a doctor recommending *only* an injection is like a mechanic slapping a piece of duct tape over your check-engine light. Because if the underlying problem is not fixed, sooner or later, something's going to blow.
- **Every single one weakens you—100 percent of the time.** The same study that found that NSAIDs hurt you also found that corticosteroid injections hinder how you heal on a microscopic level, disrupt vital chemical processes, and ultimately suppress the very function of the tissue they're used on. These authors conclude by warning that corticosteroids (and NSAIDS) are, "no longer recommended for chronic soft tissue injuries or for acute ligament injuries, except for the shortest possible time, if at all."[42]

I don't know about you, but if that is the best I can hope for, then count me out. What boggles my mind—and I hope you also see the insanity behind it—is that despite all the evidence against injections, they're still given every day. Why? Maybe it's because insurance companies are still willing to pay for them, which means less out-of-pocket expense for we consumers. Maybe it's the want of getting out of pain now, and the hope it can be done in a single, in-and-out procedure. Or maybe it's that hospitals and clinics are caught in their old habits.

Who knows?

After all, if the injection didn't work, don't worry. There's plenty more where that came from.

A Dime a Dozen

Technology is great, isn't it? We can talk to a loved one across the country in an instant. All the information the world has ever created is a click away. We have TV, running water, air conditioning, and airplanes. In a lot of ways technology has bettered our lives. It has not, however, bettered your chances of getting rid of nagging back and neck pain.

More and more procedures are being developed that harness the power of technology to propel people out of pain. The pain industry has been climbing this ladder of "technological advances" for years, and can now do things that were once thought impossible. This is fine except for one very important, very crucial thing: for back and neck pain, the ladder is leaning against the wrong wall. Before I describe this fundamental flaw, here are some examples of other techie, and mostly disappointing, invasive procedures.

- **DENERVATION a.k.a. NERVE KILLING:** It's exactly as it sounds. Doctors use alcohol, scalpels, or lasers, with the assistance of advanced imaging, to kill nerves that detect pain. At best, it's somewhat helpful in the short term. In the long term, when you cut through a nerve, you injure it, so *when* (not *if*) it grows back, it is damaged and sensitized, which means more pain in the long run.
- **PAIN PUMPS:** A doctor inserts a pump under the skin, runs a catheter from the pump to the low back, and programs the pump to deliver pain-numbing medications. Of course, with any surgery, there's risk, but once the pump is inserted, there's the added risk, albeit small, of the catheter kinking, tearing, leaking, and causing drug overdose or under dose. [43]
- **ELECTRIC STIMULATION:** This is a techie way to trick the brain not to feel pain. By electrically stimulating non-pain nerves, the brain is prevented from feeling pain from the pain nerves. This procedure has many names: Transcutaneous Electrical Nerve Stimulation (TENS), Peripheral Nerve Field Stimulation (PNFS), Spinal Cord Stimulation (SCS), and Deep Brain Stimulation (DBS). Each one is more invasive than the last and brings with it more risk.

None of these work for everyone, and all of these—as well as injections and medications—are based on a myth that has led to the dismay and suffering of millions. This myth is the fundamental flaw I was talking about earlier.

Let me tell you a short story to illustrate the point.

Turn Off the Faucet

On the verge of retirement, a school custodian is training his replacement. One day, right before the lunch bell, they walk into the cafeteria and are shocked to see that the floor is covered in water.

The newbie grabs a mop and bucket and frantically starts mopping. He looks up to see the soon-to-be retiree leisurely walking away.

"What are you doing? I need your help!"

Without a glance in the direction of the trainee, the old custodian turns a corner, disappearing from view.

"He must know where some better mops are," thought the young custodian as he surveyed the water-covered landscape before him. "We're gonna need them if there's any chance of cleaning up this mess before lunch." Moments later, he sees the old custodian reemerge empty-handed.

The young apprentice's face turns red and a vein pops out in his forehead as he shouts, "What on earth were you doing? I'm over here toiling away while you're acting like you're on a Sunday morning stroll!"

With a look of wisdom, the old custodian grabs the remaining mop and with a half-grin says, "You have to turn off the leaking faucet before you can clean up the mess."

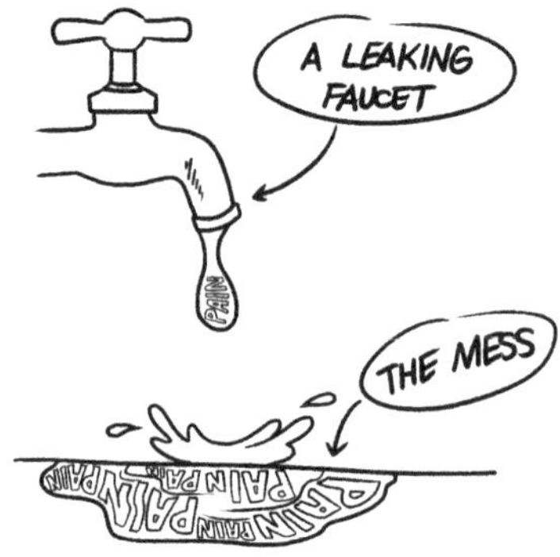

The Leaking Faucet of Pain

Pain is *a* mess—and it's also *the* mess. Pain is a result of something going wrong in your body, and all the interventions we've talked about so far are mops trying to clean it up. Nothing more, nothing less.

I promise you that the reason you're in pain is not because of a lack of medication or a lack of procedures. Your neck does not hurt because you are deficient in ibuprofen, nor does your lower back hurt because your injection levels are "below normal" or because you missed your mandatory, annual electric stimulation session.

Let me reiterate: Any pill, injection, or procedure is a mop, trying to clean up the mess of pain, and sometimes they are absolutely necessary. But if the problem that is actually causing the pain—the leaking faucet—isn't fixed, you will never, ever be pain-free. There's no getting around that fact. The pain industry, drug giants, and apparently many doctors and healthcare professionals, either don't understand or refuse to recognize this. That's why more people are suffering from pain than ever before: the approach to eliminating pain has been one-sided.

Here's the good news: I'm going tell you exactly what can be causing your back and neck pain. In Section 4 of this book, you'll learn about "The Vicious Cycle." I know you'll have a "Eureka!" moment as you read it.

Summary

- **MYTH:** *"In pain? Yeah, there's a procedure for that."* One can do a lot of things to find relief: injections, denervation, pain pumps, and electric stimulation, to name a few. Many of them might even be considered "good options" and provide temporary relief.

- **TRUTH:** None of them are the right option in and of themselves. That designation is reserved for the treatment that actually addresses whatever problem is causing the pain.

Chapter 8

MYTH 6: The Spinal Surgery Debacle—"Surgery Is Your Best Option"

The rapid and enthusiastic expansion of disc surgery soon exposed its limitations and failures. It was accused of leaving more tragic human wreckage in its wake than any other operation in history.
—Allan & Waddell, *A Historical Perspective On Low Back Pain and Disability,* 1989

Surgery is the sacred cow of our health-care system and surgeons are the sacred cowboys who milk it.
—David Spodick, MD, professor at the University of Massachusetts

Whether you like it or not, if you're in pain long enough, eventually you'll find yourself in a surgeon's office. It's there that some pain sufferers are told to go under the knife because it's their best option for relief. Others are told that it's their only option. It's all a *lie*. The truth is that surgery is the worst option, period.

What pain sufferers aren't told is that by trying to cut out the pain, they're really cutting away their only chance of ever becoming pain-free. Let me show you why.

Spinal Fusions

The idea behind a spinal fusion is not complicated: if a spinal joint is causing trouble, bind it to the good joints neighboring it. That way, it can't be trouble anymore. When fusions first arrived on the scene, they were touted as the *perfect fix* for back and neck pain. It didn't take long before the number of spinal fusion procedures skyrocketed.

This was fine, except that years later, after millions of operations had been performed, one very real, very permanent problem began to surface. Many spinal surgery patients learned the hard way that however bad your back and neck was before, after a fusion it can be much worse.

In 2011, the journal *Spine* published an article where researchers reviewed records of 1,450 patients who were suffering from disc degeneration, disc herniation, or radiculopathy—a nerve condition that causes tingling, numbness, pain, or weakness in the limbs. What they found was shocking: having a spinal fusion increases the risk of being permanently disabled by *500 percent.*

That doesn't sound like a "perfect fix" to me.

These 1,450 patients were people whose pain was so bad they couldn't work, so when the researchers looked to see how many people had returned to work after spinal fusion surgery, they discovered that 74 percent of those who had the operation still weren't back to work two years later.

Not only that, they found that over a quarter of spinal fusion patients had to have additional surgeries.[44] Considering that success rates plummet to 30 percent after a second spine surgery, 15 percent after a third, and approximately 5 percent after a fourth[45], you may start to wonder why spinal fusions are done at all. That's a good question with a not-so-nice answer. But before I tell you what it is, let's look at the other kind of spinal surgery.

–Ectomy: Suffix Meaning "The Surgical Removal of"

Instead of fusing segments, the other form of spinal surgery involves cutting away parts of the spine in the hope of relieving pain. Here are the most common types:

- ✓ **Disc-ectomy:** When a piece of your intervertebral disc (spinal cushion) gets chopped off. Usually done when there's a herniation or bulged disc.
- ✓ **Lamin-ectomy:** When bone located on the back part of the spinal column is removed. Usually due to a disc problem or degeneration.
- ✓ **Foramin-ectomy:** When bone or tissue clogging the passageway for the nerve gets drilled clean.

While this type of spinal surgery may (or may not) temporarily relieve pain, in the long run, it eats away at your spine like rust on a car, and that fact is often not emphasized when the surgery option is being discussed. This erosion of the spine has a name:

Transitional Syndrome/Adjacent Segment Disease

To understand this, you'll need a crash course on the back and neck. So sit up straight and pay attention. Your spine is a repeating chain of vertebrae and cartilage. Each segment works with the neighboring segments to absorb stress brought on by sitting, bending, lifting, etc. This is important because by each piece absorbing a little, no one piece has to absorb a lot—an essential process to having a pain-free back and neck.

Surgery disrupts this.

When you cut through muscles and ligaments and cut out cartilage and bone, that specific spot ceases to do its part of absorbing stress. When one part of the chain does not work properly, the stress gets transferred or "transitions" somewhere else—the neighboring joints.

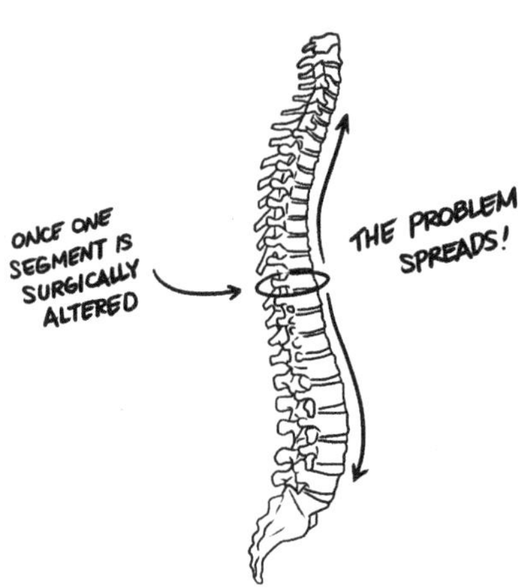

Where once the problem was limited to one, two, or maybe three areas, now it spreads like an infection up and down the entire spine. Bone spurs grow like weeds, discs tear and herniate, the passageways for nerves get clogged, and arthritis runs rampant.[47]

You see, this "transference" takes place after spinal surgery in which a neck or back problem goes to other places. If it goes to adjacent segments of the spine, it's called Adjacent Segment Disease. If it goes to the extremities (shoulders, arms, hips, and legs) it's called Transitional Syndrome. It may take months or years, but no matter how skilled the surgeon is—it is not a question of *if* this happens, but only a matter of *when* and *how badly* it happens.

Believe it or not, that's actually the best-case scenario. There are some cases where pain doesn't transition at all. It actually never leaves.

Failed Back Surgery Syndrome

What is it? It is just as it sounds. A person goes into surgery and comes out with the same level of pain or worse. Bluntly said, the operation didn't work.

Be careful not to let the simplicity of the name undersell its meaning. Have you ever heard of "failed heart-surgery syndrome"? "Failed kidney-surgery syndrome"? Or "failed knee-surgery syndrome"? No, you haven't, because they don't exist. Failed Back Surgery Syndrome isn't a random slang term christened by an upset patient. It is an official diagnosis handed down from medical regulators. This disturbingly poor outcome has happened to thousands of people over years that eventually it *had* to be recognized. That's a lot of necks, backs, and lives ruined.

> ***"The world of spinal medicine, unfortunately, is producing patients with failed back surgery syndrome at an alarming rate."***
> **—July 2004 "The Back Letter" (a newsletter from the Department of Orthopedic Surgery at Georgetown Medical Center in Washington, DC)**

No other type of surgery in the world has an actual diagnosis due to its history of poor results...that award goes to spinal surgery alone.

Another Nail in the Coffin

A study conducted in 1999, and published in the *Journal of Bone and Joint Surgery,* took an interesting approach to the problem of spinal surgery. Researchers compared regions where they were doing a lot of spinal surgeries to those doing only a few. This is what they found: the best outcomes for back pain occurred where surgery rates were lowest, and the worst results occurred in areas where surgery rates were highest.[47] What does that mean? Wherever and whenever spinal surgery is performed the most, the chances of getting rid of pain is the worst!

We could end this chapter here, but the whole story hasn't been told yet.

A Deep Cut

According to a 2005 study titled "Evidence-Informed Management of Chronic Low Back Pain." outside of serious structural disease like an infection, tumor, or such severe spinal deterioration that your life is at risk, there are no clear guidelines telling doctors to perform spinal surgery to relieve back pain.[48] Zero. None. Nada. Zilch.

While this may be news to you, this has been known in the medical community for quite some time. But guess what's happening? Despite an epidemic of failed spinal surgeries, people are still going under the knife and doing it in large numbers.

Between the years 1992–2007, Medicare spending on spinal surgeries more than doubled.[49] In 2012, over a *million* spinal surgeries were performed across the nation officially making it the most common type of surgery.[50]

This isn't going unnoticed. Many people "in the know" realize something isn't right. One group of researchers said that, "There remains little or no medical, clinical, or surgical evidence to support such variability."[49] Don't breeze by that statement. They're saying that there really isn't any evidence that justifies all of these spine surgeries being performed.

Why are they still being done so often?

The nice answer: Our aging population is plainly more willing to accept spinal surgery as a good option because they're trying to stay active.

The not-so-nice answer: The spinal surgery industry has become more about the bottom line than your neck and back.

Cut to the Chase

How has money—that is literally coming off the backs of pain sufferers—become a driving force for spinal surgery?

- ✓ **Surgeons get paid more for doing more complex surgeries.** It only makes sense. The more difficult the surgery, the more a surgeon *should* get paid for his skills. The problem is that these more complex surgeries are being performed when simpler, less expensive, and just as effective options are available. Richard Deyo, pain researcher, notes that *possibly up to 50 percent of these more complex surgeries being done are unnecessary.*[51] That's more than just a few over-zealous surgeons.
- ✓ **The hardware used is a goldmine.** "You can easily put $30,000 into a person during a fusion surgery," notes Charles Rosen, spine surgeon at University of California who created a group to combat what it sees as conflicts of interest in spine surgery. What kind of profit margins are the manufacturers of spine surgery hardware looking at? Consider this: the screws used to drill into bone, called pedicle screws, can be manufactured for less than $100 and are sold for $1000 to $2000 apiece.[52]

That's a lot of profit.

✓ **Physician-owned distributorships.** This is a business that a doctor is an investor in, and distributor of, the devices or hardware he may put into his patients. While it is a legal arrangement, the Department of Health and Human Services' Office of Inspector General has concluded that these distributorships are "inherently suspect," and issued fraud alerts in 2006 and 2013.[53]

You're probably reeling from all of this information. It's shocking I know, but it's true. It's equally true that there are some fine spine surgeons who operate (in every sense of the word) with honesty and integrity, using all of the skills and experience they have acquired. And they have nothing but their patients' best interests at heart. Having said that, it seems there are some bad apples in the bunch, but you're now armed with some vital information to help you make informed decisions about your own health.

The Final Cut

In her book, *A Nation in Pain,* author Judy Foreman got it right when she wrote, "The majority of surgery patients do not have an optimal outcome. That is, having minimal-to-no pain, reduction of pain medications, and a return to high-level functioning."

Every time a new patient comes to my office, and on their intake form, they have checked "yes" to having had spinal surgery, I'm reminded of this pain myth, all the people it's affected, and the simple truth behind it.

Summary

- **MYTH:** *Spinal surgery is your best or only option for pain relief.*

Two peas in a pod. Spinal fusions bind joints together while "ectomies" remove pieces of the spine, both in the hope of relieving pain. While they can help in cases of severe instability, infection, or a tumor, for back and neck pain their track record is terrible.

Cut in and cut away. By cutting into the spine, you disrupt its ability to absorb stress, and doing so ultimately leads to more problems and potentially much more pain.

The power of money. There are financial incentives for surgeons and hospitals to operate that is undoubtedly linked to the massive number of spinal surgeries being performed.

- **TRUTH:** Spinal surgery is the worst option when it comes to relieving back and neck pain and should only be considered when all other avenues have been thoroughly exhausted, if at all.

Chapter 9

Myth 7: The Magic Bullet

There are no magic bullets for chronic back pain, and expecting a cure… is generally wishful thinking"[1]
—Richard Deyo, M.D., pain researcher

Leeches.

What comes to your mind when you read that word? Gross? Slimy? Blood suckers? What if I told you the pain industry is full of leeches? And that every year new ones enter the water hungry to feast on pain sufferers? But they aren't out for blood. These leeches are only interested in draining you of your hard-earned money.

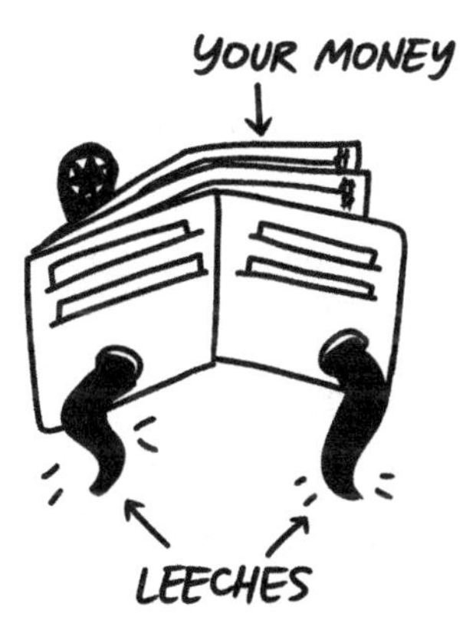

They come in different shapes, sizes, and prices, but they are all selling the same thing: A magic bullet—a remedy that promises to get rid of back and neck pain once and for all.

Don't fall for their lies.

As Seen on TV

One of the things pain interferes with most *is rest*. It makes it hard to fall asleep and even more difficult to stay asleep. When you're tired and frustrated because your neck, back, shoulder, or leg pain has forced you up again—that's when the leeches swarm.

Here's the setup.

You turn on the TV and a B-list celebrity introduces an expert who walks onstage, applauded by a bought-and-paid-for audience. This guru has developed a little known "cure-all" that will get rid of your pain. Suddenly, the TV cuts to a testimonial; a middle-aged person who looks a lot like someone you know. She says something like, "I've tried everything, spent tons of money, and nothing worked. I used the guru's trick and now I'm pain-free. And you can be too!"

This cycle of forced enthusiasm, applause, rehearsed questions, and over-the-top testimonials repeats a few times before a smooth voice chimes in, "If you act now you can save not $25, not $50, but $100! But wait there's more. All of this for three easy payments of $XX.99. There's a 90-day, money-back guarantee so if you're not completely satisfied, send it back, no extra charge. Call now!"

Sound familiar?

This sales recipe has been used for years. Here's list of magic bullets you may have seen in the past:

- Lie down, put your legs on this machine, and it will do

all the work. It opens up the joints and loosens up nasty muscle knots. Once you own this device, your back pain will never stop you from living life to the fullest.

- The amazing flip-upside-down table that decompresses your back. Look at their smiles as they hang upside down. No way can they be in pain if they're that happy. You'll wonder how you've been able to live without it once you've tried it!
- Wear this magnet that polarizes your blood and gets rid of back and neck pain instantly!
- The wrap with unique pressure pads that apply specific pressure to targeted areas. When you wear it, you'll feel 20 years younger!
- The new supplement filled with just-discovered berries from the heart of the African rain forest, which fill the joints full of nutrients that kill pain!
- The shoe insert, made with special material, that eliminate posture problems, and back pain, leg pain, and foot pain.
- The device that looks like a garage door opener that uses fast-acting infrared light and laser therapy to soothe pain and stiffness out of your muscles and joints.

Missing the Mark

As you can see, there's no shortage of magic bullets. Isn't that odd? Why do new magic bullets keep getting invented? You would think that if they are doing their job, we wouldn't need new ones.

But that's not what's happening.

People keep buying these products because they're still in pain. And they're still in pain because these magic bullets have the same fundamental flaw that medications, invasive procedures, and spinal surgery have: they're a mop, and they don't turn off the faucet. No device, contraption, potion, lotion, or pill will ever fix back and neck pain, and the only thing a magic bullet remedies is the salesman's empty wallet. That's the truth.

A Wake-up Call

A little known fact about the Golden Gate Bridge is that it's always being painted. As soon as the painters have completed a coat, they start again, putting on another one. It's a never-ending work in progress. For many, getting and staying as pain-free as possible is like that.

Back and neck pain is not like a cut on your finger where you treat it, it heals, and you never have to think about it again. Instead it's like heart disease or diabetes where you treat it, it improves, and then you do what is necessary in order to stop it from coming back.

Now, I need to make something very clear about my message because it could be taken the wrong way. Just because back and neck pain is not "fixable"—meaning that once it's gone, it's gone forever—it does not mean you're destined to suffer from pain forever. Getting your back and neck pain-free, or as close to it as possible, is very doable. The key is that once the pain is relieved; you need to "stabilize" it so that it stays that way. Very specific things must be done to accomplish that—and this is what "The Solution" is all about. It's not a magic bullet, cure-all, or "one-and-done" way to get rid of pain that you will want to replace in a few months. It is a fundamentally different approach using principles that have withstood the test of time, as well as scientific scrutiny.

Another One Bites the Dust

We have pulled back the curtains on yet another pain myth. I hope the smoke is beginning to clear, and you're seeing the pain industry in its true form. Soon, we will be exploring the commonly misunderstood purpose of pain, how it develops in the back and neck (called The Vicious Cycle), the exciting research on the most effective approach to eliminating pain, and most importantly, how to turn off "the pain faucet" once and for all.

But first, we have two more myths to bust.

Summary

- **MYTH:** There is a magic bullet that cures back and neck pain.

    Leeches. Every year there is a new product on the market boasting its ability to cure your pain. Don't fall for it. These products are here one day and gone the next because they don't address the cause of back and neck pain.

    Stable vs. Fixed. Back and neck pain, especially chronic back and neck pain, is like diabetes, heart disease, or asthma. While not necessarily "fixable," it can be dramatically improved. Once they're "stable," the focus changes to keeping them that way.

    An apple a day. Like maintaining a healthy smile, keeping the back and neck pain-free takes some thought and effort every day. Much like brushing your teeth, but for your spine.

- **TRUTH:** The only thing a *magic bullet* cures is the salesman's empty wallet. To have your back and neck go from being painful to being pain-free, you must get to the root of the problem (turn off the faucet). More on this later.

Chapter 10

MYTH 8: "Learn to Live with It"

I was in constant pain. I couldn't think. I couldn't function. My family was falling apart. I didn't know what to do.
—Carl White, father, chronic pain sufferer

People who aren't in constant pain don't understand the toll it takes. There's more to the experience than just the never-ending push-you-to-your-limits pain. Pain diminishes life. It depletes bank accounts, devastates relationships, and limits potential. And when you've tried anything and everything to get relief, and you're still in pain, it's easy to believe you're going to have to learn to live with it.

The tricky thing about this "You-Have-to-Live-With-It" myth is that its real message is obscured. Let me show you:

✓ **It's an incomplete sentence.** The full message is, "You're going to have to learn to live with the pain *because this is as good as it's going to get.*" It means your best days are behind you and it's all downhill from here. Until you take your last breath, this pain will remain a big part of your life.

✓ **It's sugar-coated.** Learn to live with pain? Hardly. You'll never learn to live with pain. It doesn't work that way. *At best, you put up with suffering through it.* Not being able to play with your kids—that's suffering through it. Not being able to go for a walk—that's suffering through it. Not being able to sleep a full night—that's suffering through it. When we start to believe this lie, we accept not only the sensation of pain as a part of our life, but also all of the restrictions, limitations, and lack-of-life that comes with it.

Laid bare, the real message is: "*You're just going to have to suffer through it because this is as good as it's going to get.*" And it's the first myth of this kind. All the myths up to this point entice you with the possibility of getting better, but this one is the opposite. It leads you to believe there's no hope and no end in sight for your misery. That's enough to cause fear in even the toughest pain sufferer.

Before I reveal the truth behind this myth, let's uncover how it leads to one of the most dangerous and hard-to-get-rid-of habits that will keep you in pain: *fear-avoidance behaviors.*

Force of Habit

As humans, we are hardwired to avoid pain. When we do something that causes pain, we quickly develop fear around doing that thing again. In most cases, like touching a hot iron, this is good because it protects us from injury, but with back and neck pain, it's a different story.

Your spine requires stress to stay strong, movement to stay mobile, and activity to keep you pain-free. If every time you vacuum, your back is thrown into thunderous spasms, you're going to avoid vacuuming for as long as possible. That's where the problem starts because vacuuming stresses your back and that stimulation keeps it strong. The same could be said for just about an activity that involves moving your back and neck throughout the day. So if you stop vacuuming, you stop stressing your back, and by doing so, your back will grow weak, which leads to more pain. For someone in constant pain, where the slightest thing causes pain, this turns into a very sticky mess.

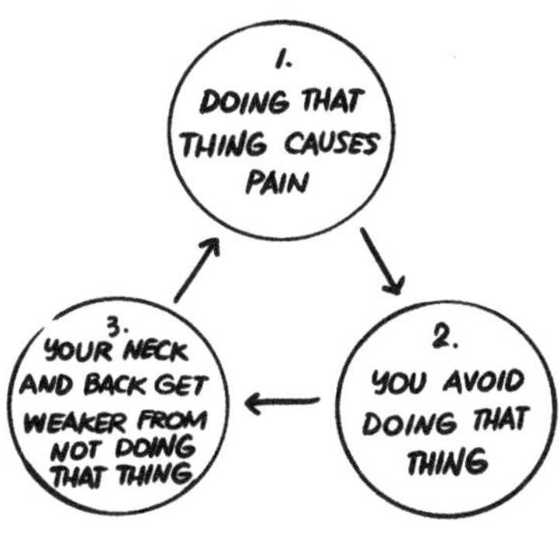

Everyday activities get increasingly difficult, and as a result of this, we avoid doing more, which causes more weakness, more pain…and soon the fear of doing things spreads to other areas of your life, as does the pain. One author put it this way: "*Pain-related fear leads to a cycle of decreased movement, inflammation, nervous system sensitization, and further decreased mobility.*"[54]

Another way to think about it: engineers tell us that if our car sits out in the driveway, it will rust faster than it will wear out cruising the open roads. It's true that if you drive a car eventually it will break down and need to be repaired—but that doesn't stop you from driving, does it? Of course not. We all know that's a part of the deal. It's the same thing with pain: you can't let it stop you from using your body; not using it will cause it to breakdown so much faster than it should, and you'll be a lot worse off.

And that's why this myth is so dangerous. If you believe that your back and neck pain is as good as it's going to get, you are also going to believe there's no point in trying to get it to improve. These beliefs go hand-in-hand with each other. And if you surrender and start doing less, you will become weaker and forced to suffer through the agony of more pain.

I've worked with people firsthand where this cycle has progressed so far, and their pain has become so bad that they don't feel life is worth living any more.

Don't give into this myth—it's a lie.

The truth is that there is *always* potential for your back and neck pain to improve. *Always.* You might have problems with your spine—and if you're reading this, they're probably big problems—but that does *not* mean you have to suffer the rest of your life.

At the end of this book, you're going to have a big epiphany when you learn the "Five Daily Habits"—especially when you learn how easy they are to make a part of your routine. These habits will keep you from developing these "avoidance behaviors" because they do one thing: make your spine healthier by improving how you use it. I'm excited to share these insights with you, but before we do—you guessed it—we have another myth to bust, our last.

Summary

- **MYTH:** "You're as good as you're going to get. It's best if you just learn to live with the pain." This myth is a full-frontal attack on the most important characteristic of getting pain-free: hope.
- **TRUTH:** You can never get as good as you're going to get, and if you surrender and *"learn to live with pain,"* you begin down a slippery slope that leads to more pain. You can always do something to improve. In fact, I'll prove it to you

right now. Did you know that a small study in 2001 showed that monosodium glutamate (MSG)—a flavor enhancer found in everything from ranch dressing to fast-food restaurant meat—causes pain nerves (nociceptors) to become sensitized? And that people who eliminated it from their diet for four consecutive months all but *eliminated* their chronic pain symptoms?[55] I'm guessing you didn't know that. I'm guessing no doctor or guru has told you that. But that's what I mean when I say there is always something you can do to improve. Don't give up. Keep reading.

Chapter 11

Myth 9: The Normal Myth— "This Type of Thing is Normal"

Be sure to put your feet in the right place, then stand firm.
—Abraham Lincoln, 16th president of the U.S.

Okay, let's get real. *Pain is everywhere, and if you're not suffering from it, I guarantee that you know someone who is.* Nearly 100 million Americans suffer from back and neck pain.[56] Which means that for every man, woman, and child you know, one in three is experiencing pain. This number is continuing to grow, with no end in sight.

That's not all.

Between 1987 and 2013, the cost of treating back pain in the U.S. ballooned 538 percent to a whopping $42.5 billion.[57] If you combine that with other pain complaints like headaches, shoulder, hip, and knee pain, then Americans spend more money on pain remedies—and lose more money because of pain—than the economy of Norway generates in a year. We're talking upwards of $350 billion[58]—that's $11,000 per second. Pain is costing a lot of people a great deal of money.

However, this is only the tip of the iceberg.

Because we've been in an uncontained epidemic of pain for decades, most of us have come to believe that back and neck pain is a normal part of life. It's not. The truth is that the line between what's normal and what's common has become so blurred that we can't tell the difference anymore. But not for much longer because we are going to boldly redraw that line, get back in touch with reality, and from there, take our first steps toward becoming pain-free.

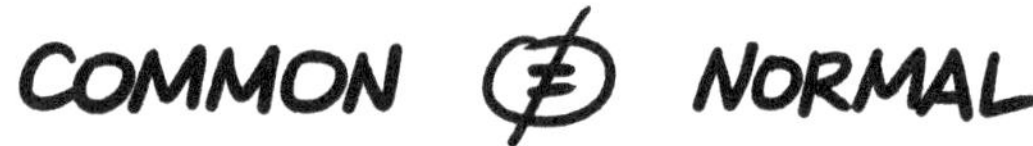

The End of the Line

Here's the shortlist of what's believed to be normal, but really isn't.

- **The older I get, the more I'll hurt, and the less I'll do.** Doing what I do affords me a unique perspective on the relationship between pain and age. The oldest patient at my clinic is ninety-two. She drives, gardens, cooks, and golfs nine holes every Wednesday. Does she experience pain? Yes. Does it stop her from living? No. On the other hand, I've worked with teenagers who can hardly get out of bed in the morning because of pain. Are they experiencing pain? Yes. Does it stop them from living? Absolutely. The truth is that pain doesn't care how old you are. It can strike whether you're a spring chicken or in your golden years because age is not what determines whether or not you're in pain. The determining factor is how well you are using your body, and the more years that pass means more opportunities to either help or hurt your back and neck.

How can you tell if you've been doing a good job with your spine? Let's go to the next item on our list.

- **Arthritis is due to aging.** I think we all can agree that a person in their twenties is not old. Yet, a 2015 study showed that up to 40 percent of young people today already have spine cartilage deterioration—a hallmark of spinal arthritis.[59] When you combine this with the fact that joints are designed to last about 110 years, it should make you wonder why so many people think that aging causes arthritis. Maybe it's because every day, while pointing to an X-ray, doctors tell patients that their pain and stiffness is due to arthritis, and "you know, this is simply a part of getting older." Here's a health insight: X-rays and MRIs do not tell us how good our joints are, but rather how good we are at using our joints. And when you use your back and neck improperly, the joints get inflamed and start deteriorating—a.k.a. arthritis. The truth is: *arthritis is not a measurement of age, it's a measurement of the amount of times you've used that joint improperly.*

You may be wondering if we're going to tackle pain in the younger years of life. I'm sure you've heard that…

- **Growing pains are a normal part of childhood.** The Mayo Foundation of Research and Information finds that there is no evidence that childhood growth should be painful or that growing pains are even related to growth. "The cause of growing pain is unknown. But there is no evidence that a child's growth is painful. And growing pains don't usually happen where growth is occurring or during times of rapid growth."[60] But, once again, because it's so common, most parents don't hesitate to chalk up their child's latest complaint to the pains of growing up. Is it possible a larger and overlooked problem is leaving kids in this misery?

And last but not least…

- **It runs in the family.** "My grandma had it. My mom has it. Now I have it." The belief that pain gets passed on like an unwanted hand-me-down is one of the oldest myths, and also one of the toughest to uproot. To see this in a new light, we need only think of the old "Nature vs. Nurture" debate. The nature side argues that our health is a result of our inherited genes. The nurture side argues that our health is mostly dependent on the environment in which we're raised. You don't hear much about it anymore because the argument was settled: they both are involved, but "Nurture" is, by far, the biggest influencer. And so it is with back and neck pain. The bony framework you inherited from your parents plays a role in your ability to live a pain-free life, but it's certainly not the lead role. That spotlight belongs to how we learn to use our back and neck. You see, the truth is we acquire much of how we move (walking, bending, dancing, lifting, etc.), and our postural habits (how you care for your spine on a daily basis), from watching those closest to us: our families. And unless you're lucky enough to have had parents who were extraordinarily ahead of their time and understood the dynamics of proper spine usage, chances are you don't know how to move properly, and thus you haven't acquired the needed postural habits to be pain-free.

In this list of what's commonly believed to be normal, but really isn't, how many items have crept into your way of thinking?

True North

The point of this chapter was to draw a line between *what's normal* and *what's common.*

- It's common to have recurring low-back pain, but it's never normal.
- It's common to "carry your stress" in your shoulders, but it's never normal.
- It's common to have tight hamstrings, degenerating discs, headaches during menses, and stubborn muscle knots, but it's never, ever, normal.

Summary

- **MYTH:** *This type of thing is normal.*
  - **A lot of people are hurting.** Research indicates that one in three Americans is dealing with pain at this very moment. And I believe that number is low.
  - **A lot of money is being spent on pain.** $42.5 billion per year. $11,000 per second. Think of what it would do for our economy and our nation, if that money was being put to better use.
- **TRUTH:** Because pain is so widespread, we've lost our bearings on what's normal for the back and neck and what's common. And so, like hikers without a compass and map,

pain sufferers often end up lost in attempting to get to their desired destination—a pain-free life. But not for much longer.

Chapter 12

A Brief Break (Summary of Section 2)

All truths are easy to understand once they are discovered; the point is to discover them.—Galileo Galilei, astronomer

Increases in the rates of imaging, opioid prescriptions, injections, and fusion surgery might be justified if there were substantial improvements in patient outcomes; unfortunately, they do not. In fact, statistics indicate that disability from musculoskeletal disorders is rising, not falling.—"Over-treating Chronic Back Pain: Time of Back Off?" *Journal of the American Board of Family Medicine*

We have covered a lot of ground. Let's recap the myths we have shattered, and the truths we have uncovered thus far. We have learned that:

- Big Pharma spends a lot of time, energy, and money trying to get you to believe that their medications are the answer for your pain. They aren't. Pain meds have dangerous side effects and many of them, including the ones we're told it's okay to take daily, are downright deadly.

- Most doctors *do* have your best interests in mind, but that *doesn't* change the fact that Big Pharma puts an extraordinary amount of pressure on them in order to influence their recommendations. The sharp increase in pain medication usage over the past few years is evidence that their marketing efforts are working. So while most doctors certainly do have your best interests in mind, it may not be the only thing on their mind.
- Invasive procedures are fundamentally flawed. They treat pain without treating *the cause* of pain. This leads to short-lived results with long-term consequences.
- Remember what author Judy Foreman said, "The majority of surgery patients do not have an optimal outcome. That is, having minimal-to-no pain, reduction of pain medications, and a return to high-level functioning." Certainly, when it comes to back and neck pain, patients need to consider long and hard if surgery is *really* their best option.
- Salesmen with their latest and greatest "magic bullets" are here to stay and the only thing their cure-alls remedy is the own empty wallets. The body isn't something that gets "fixed." It is something that gets as good as possible, and then we have to work to keep it there. That's how it is with pain, too.
- You never really learn to live with pain. You're forced to suffer through it. Most important though, if you buy into this self-defeating belief, the pain avoidance habits you develop will make your suffering worsen as time goes on.
- Lastly, *normal* and *common* are not the same thing. A lot of people are hurting, but this doesn't make it normal.

> We're not supposed to hurt more as we age. Aging doesn't cause arthritis. There's no proof that growing pains are a normal part of childhood. And lastly, your genes play only a small role in your ability to be pain-free.

Has the blindfold been removed from your eyes? Are you beginning to see clearly now? Are you viewing the pain industry any differently? Right now, we are laying the foundations for getting pain-free. And if these myths are alarming or disturbing to you, good! That's exactly what I felt. I let those feelings motivate me to dig deeper and figure out "The Solution" to back and neck pain, and I hope you'll let everything you've learned so far fuel your desire to follow "The Solution" and get yourself pain-free. Before I tell you what's coming next, first let me say a couple things.

Putting My Cards on the Table

From what I have written so far, you might assume that I am anti-medications, surgery, and doctors. But that's not the case. Let me tell you why. When I was eight years old, I was in an accident. I popped a wheelie while riding on a dock, lost my balance, and fell directly onto a blunt post. Many of my ribs had been fractured, my diaphragm torn, my spleen ruptured, and I was bleeding internally. I was emergency airlifted to a children's hospital, and was in intensive care for weeks. Many times the doctors and my parents thought I was going to die. The tremendous skill of doctors and staff using drugs and surgery saved my life. It's because of doctors, medications, and surgery that I am here and able to write this book today.

I love medications, surgery, and doctors when they are absolutely necessary, and are used at the right time for the right reasons. As we all should. But I *do not* love medication, surgery, and doctors when they are not necessary and used at the wrong time and for the wrong reasons—especially for back and neck pain.

I have no problem with Big Pharma, surgeons, doctors, and hospitals making a lot of money by prescribing medications and performing surgery. I believe they should be paid for their work. And if they're good at what they do, they should be paid well—*but only if the treatment is safe and effective.*

I have a big problem with people making money off pain sufferers when treatment is unsafe and ineffective. I think it's sick. I think it's wrong. I think it needs to stop, and I hope what you've read so far has caused a righteous anger to stir within you because that's what's needed if things are ever going to change.

Time to Wrap It Up

Take a deep breath. In fact, put down the book, stand up, and do some good stretching. Go ahead. I'll still be here when you come back.

You're back? Great.

With these myths exposed for what they really are—disempowering beliefs that leave you helpless, hopeless, and most importantly *still in pain*—we are going to take another step closer to being pain-free.

If you're the type of person who wants to get to the point and learn "The Solution" to back and neck pain, skip to Section 5. For the rest of us, our next step is learning the basics of pain, nerves, muscles, and joints. And then, I'm going to introduce you to the culprit of back and neck pain: The Vicious Cycle.

Let's get started.

SECTION 3

Learning The Basics

The minute you get away from fundamentals, whether it's proper technique, work ethic, or mental preparation, the bottom can fall out of your game, your schoolwork, your job, whatever you're doing.

—Michael Jordan, professional basketball player,
winner of six NBA championships

Chapter 13

The Basics: Pain

When the body sends us a message in the form of pain, we should make sense out of it, rather than numb our senses to it.
—Dr. F. H. Barge

Nowadays it seems that nearly everyone on the planet knows what a car is. In America, most of us own one or two. We've grown up around them, we've been on car trips, we've taken classes and passed tests to drive them, and through all of that, we've learned the basics of owning and operating a car like:

- Look behind you while in reverse.
- If the gas gauge is low, fill up your tank.
- If the check engine light comes on, bring it in to the mechanic.
- A yellow light means slow down and yield.

The list goes on and on. And though most of us understand these basics, very few of us could explain the dynamics of the internal combustion engine despite it being the very thing that makes a car a car. If you think about it, it takes no knowledge to own a car, and little knowledge to drive one.

Pain is very similar…

A lot of people are in pain, and it's nearly impossible not to have at least some contact with pain in your day-to-day life. You don't need to understand pain in order to suffer from it, and you certainly don't need to explain the complex biochemistry behind pain in order to feel it. You do, however, need to know the basics of pain in order to have as little pain as possible in your life.

And that's what we're going to cover next.

The Basics: A Canary in a Coal Mine

What do you suppose the purpose of pain is? To make your life uncomfortable? To get in your way? To stop you from having fun? To remind you that you're getting older?

Of course not.

At the turn of the 20th century, carbon monoxide poisoning was one of the deadliest threats facing coal miners. You see, carbon monoxide gas forms as a result of the incomplete combustion of a fuel. While mining coal, which is a fuel, if there was a fire or an explosion, carbon monoxide gas would form and accumulate within the mine. This was a big problem because carbon monoxide gas, as you probably know, is odorless, tasteless, invisible—and deadly. As none of their senses could detect it, miners wouldn't know they were poisoned until it was too late.

Then along came a scientist who discovered what causes carbon monoxide poisoning and suggested that, because canaries are highly sensitive to toxic gases, miners should carry them down into the mines to serve as an early-warning system. As the miners were toiling away, if they saw a dead canary, it meant that they themselves were being poisoned. This warning sign bought miners precious moments and saved lives.

What does this history lesson have to do with pain?

As a dead canary was a warning sign for miners, pain is a warning sign for you.

But a warning sign of what? The answer is found in the word "pain" itself.

The word pain comes from the Latin "poena," meaning penalty. In a way, pain means that your body is paying the penalty—which is bodily damage. When something damages the body, specialized nerves called nociceptors (remember them?) send signals to the brain, which the brain then translates into the sensation of pain.

Pain, then, is your body alerting you to damage.

That answers the question of what pain is, but we haven't answered the more important question of: *why do we have pain?*

The Basics: Pain's Purpose

Imagine for a moment that you couldn't feel pain. What would life be like? Some of you are probably thinking, "Yes, please. I'll have some of that." Not so fast.

Consider leprosy.

Leprosy is an infectious disease that causes severe skin sores and nerve damage, so much so that the infected person can lose the ability to feel pain. Dr. Paul Brand, a world-renowned expert on the subject, in his book *The Gift of Pain*, warns us why not being able to feel pain is a bad thing, and alludes to what pain's purpose really is:

> "In an extreme form, this inability to 'hear' pain can cause

permanent damage because the body's careful response to danger will break down.

"For example, a healthy person nearly always falls when beginning to sprain an ankle. Perhaps you step on a loose stone or curb. As your ankle begins to twist, the lateral ligaments of the ankle endure a terrific strain. The nerve cells detecting the strain categorically order the body to take all weight off the damaged leg immediately. The thigh and calf muscles will become momentarily flaccid. But if your other, undamaged leg is off the ground taking a step, you will now have no support, and will lurch to the ground. Your body prefers falling to forcing the ankle to take weight in its twisted position. You get up feeling a fool and hoping no one was watching, but in reality you have just achieved a beautifully coordinated maneuver that saved you from a sprained ankle or worse.

"However, I recall watching a leprosy victim sprain his ankle without falling. He stepped on a loose stone, turned his ankle completely over so that the sole of his foot pointed inward, and walked on without a limp. He did not even glance at the foot he had just irreparably damaged by rupturing the left lateral ligament. *He lacked the protection of pain.* Afterward, without the support of the ligament he had ruptured, he turned his ankle again and again until eventually, due to more complications, he had to have that leg amputated." (emphasis author's)[1]

Admittedly, the example he gives is a more extreme case, but the point remains the same: ***without pain, we would be unaware of injury and devoid of the body's protective mechanisms.***

You may be thinking, "Okay, Doc, I get it. Pain has a purpose. But that doesn't make my neck or back feel any better," and you'd be right. It doesn't. But knowing this information is an important step on the way to eliminate back and neck pain once and for all.

The Basics: The Pain Threshold

When you think of a threshold, what do you think of?

The word threshold comes from a time when houses had dirt floors often covered with straw or swamp grass called "thresh." A threshold held "the thresh" inside the house—clever, huh? Because of its placement, you would have to step over it to enter or exit the home. Overtime, this word began to designate a line or barrier.

Here's a quick exercise to drive home the point: From where you're sitting now, look at the nearest door and guess how many steps it would take you to get to its threshold. Now, set this book down, check to see if your guess was right, and make sure you cross the threshold. Go ahead, do it.

How close were you?

From where I'm sitting in my office, it took me five steps before I reached my door's threshold, but it wasn't until I took the sixth step, crossing over the threshold, that I entered the hallway.

In the same way the body has a "Pain Threshold," which means that problems can develop for quite some time without any pain being present. It's only once the problem worsens to the the degree that it crosses the threshold that you will start to feel pain.

For example, something bad could have happened to you three months ago, but it was not until the underlying dysfunction and damage from that injury got so bad it crossed the pain threshold that you actually begin to feel it—as is the case in many motor vehicle accidents. Another example is you could repetitively injure back and neck over the course of three years and have no idea until, again, the pain threshold is crossed. In reality, because of your body's threshold, by the time you feel pain, the damage has already been done. Then, depending on what tissue has been damaged, the pain can range from a minor irritation to excruciating pain.

It's a good thing we all have a Pain Threshold. If every time you were impacted by something or every time you did something wrong you felt pain, life would not be very much fun. Our days would be filled with more pain than we would know what to do with.

The bad thing about having a Pain Threshold is that it can lull us into a false sense of security. Here's what I mean. Many people believe that No Pain = No Problems. They think, "If I'm not in pain right now, everything is fine in my back and neck." And while there's a chance this might be true, the odds are not in your favor. It's highly likely that you have some degree of dysfunction and damage accumulating in your spine at any given moment—like the chances are good that you have some degree of cavity forming in your teeth. So really, if you're not in pain right now, it basically means that your neck or back hasn't crossed the Pain Threshold yet, and pain is soon to come. Take a moment and study this graph and you'll see what I mean.

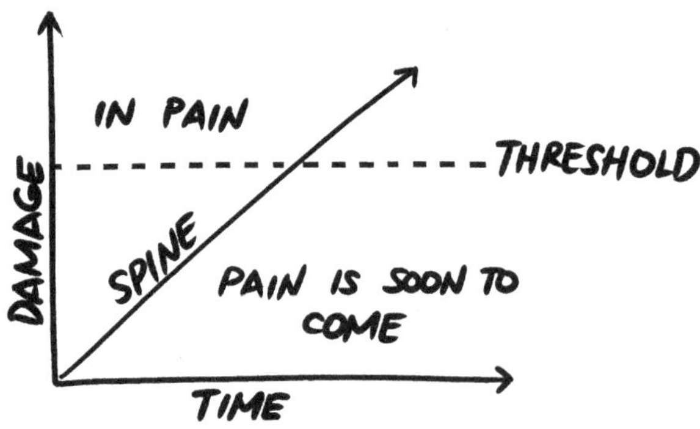

How do you know if you're headed toward trouble? Just like how there are ways to detect a cavity early, there are proven and reliable tests to detect if your neck and/or back is moving towards the Pain Threshold. I'll share one of them in the next section.

Right now, realize that it's not your responsibility to know what these tests are and how they work. Indeed, whole textbooks, classes, and degrees are focused on this subject, and only a small group of professionals have the training needed to apply them—I'm one of those people.

Your responsibility is to be aware of the Pain Threshold. and to take action when appropriate.

The Basics: Inflammation

Immediately upon being injured, the body ingeniously sets into motion a chain reaction to get you healed and out of pain. The damaged tissues release a slew of chemicals with names like "cytokines" and "interleukins," which is a good thing because these chemicals are there to protect the area, clean up the damage, and initiate healing (like calling in the fibroblasts, remember them?)

Inflammation has a bad reputation because once it's sparked, it causes redness, heat, swelling, and pain, but let's take a moment and look at the bright side.

- Redness and heat: when these occur, it means that the blood vessels have dilated, which increases the blood flow to the injured area. More blood equates to faster healing.
- Swelling: fluid accumulating around the injured area allows the "repair" cells and nutrients to stay at the site of damage. Why is this good? For the same reason a construction crew keeps their building materials close at hand—easier access

makes for a faster job. Not only that, but the swelling protects you from further injury because it eliminates excess movement.

- Pain: as we've already covered, it protects you and forces you to reckon with the problem so that you don't injure it further.

Although inflammation hurts, it is a crucial part of the healing process because it lays the groundwork the body needs in order to get out of pain. After inflammation has done its work, if everything goes according to plan, then the injured tissue will start to recover. More on this, later.

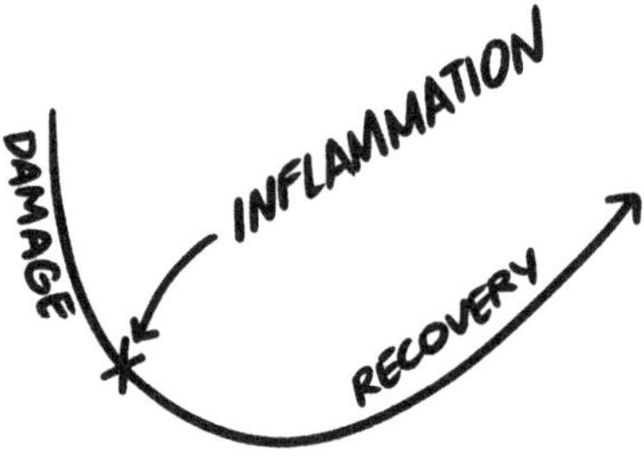

The Basics: Why Is It That Back Pain Can Be So Severe?

Have you ever wondered why back and neck pain episodes can be so severe? I remember a patient once describing to me that after bending forward, her pain was so severe that it felt like her whole body was "locked," and she couldn't move. Her coworkers had to lower her into a chair using a blanket.

What makes the spine so touchy? The spine protects the most vital part of you as a human, your central nervous system (CNS). The central nervous system is the coordinator of every other system in your body. It is considered the "master system." So, when the protective sheath of the spinal cord—vertebrae, discs, ligaments, muscles that make up the spine—are injured, your brain sees it as a serious threat, and responds accordingly to warn you about it. And it's not in a gentle whisper either. The brain is going to yell at you, making sure you understand that you've injured your spine so that you can take the appropriate steps to protect it and allow it to heal.

The Basics: When Good Pain Goes Bad

The last few paragraphs may have made sense to you, but chances are there's one hang up in the back of your mind: "Why, if pain is 'good', do I hurt so bad? Why hasn't mine gone away? How come I'm still suffering from it? Why do I still hurt?" It's as if your body has become "stuck" in pain. The wheels are spinning, but the car's not moving. Somehow, the pain that's supposed to warn you, supposed to protect you, supposed to come and then go, and supposed to *help* you is actually *hurting* you.

Why does this happen?

The reason why that one sore spot in your neck keeps showing up, or the headaches keep occurring, or the back pain won't go away, is because they're stuck in an environment that doesn't allow them to heal. You've been robbed by the greatest thief of pain-free living known to mankind—and it's something you've most likely never heard of before.

Its name? The Vicious Cycle.

We have a handful of basics regarding your nerves, muscles, and joints to cover before we dive into the Vicious Cycle, but rest assured, once we get there, you will start to see why back and neck pain can be so difficult to alleviate.

Chapter 14

The Basics: Your Nerves, Muscles, and Joints

Ignorance is not bliss. What you don't know about your body will hurt you.—Anonymous

The next few pages took an incredible amount of time to write, mostly because it's the distillation of a ton of scientific studies. If you've ever read an actual research article, you'll know the authors often use seven-dollar college words (mostly long-winded medical jargon) to "explain" their studies.

I'm not going to do that.

My goal is to present that information in such a way that you'll understand it. If I've done my job—and you pay close attention—this next part will provide the foundation necessary to understand The Vicious Cycle, and, more importantly, it will provide the springboard for you to live a pain-free life.

The Basics: Nerves, muscles, and joints are intimately connected. The term "neuromusculoskeletal system" is used to describe the close relationship that nerves, muscles, and joints have with each other. All three are absolutely essential, each serving its own unique purpose. And you can't have one without the other because they are totally integrated and have to work together. This means when something goes wrong, they all are equally damaged. Muscles move us, but the nerves coordinate such movement, and the joints provide the freedom and direction of that movement. Each element depends on the previous one, and influences the next. One of these cannot do anything, good or bad, without the next being affected by it.

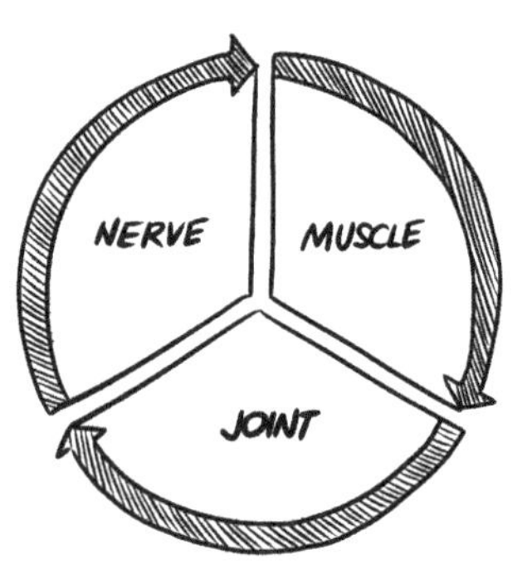

- ✓ A nerve can never react without a muscle responding.
- ✓ A muscle can never respond without a joint being affected.
- ✓ And a joint can never be affected without making a nerve react.

That's the way you're put together.

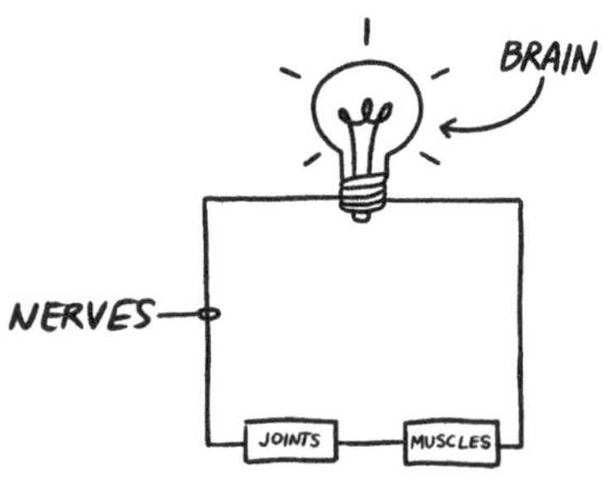

I'm going to introduce each component, and share one or two important pieces of information about how they work that will come in handy later. Remember this, though, none of these pieces were designed to become dysfunctional, damaged, and be a cause of your pain. Each was designed to do the exact opposite—to stay healthy and keep you pain-free.

The Basics: You have two types of nerves in your neuromusculoskeletal system: mechanoreceptors and nociceptors. (mek-a-no-re-sep-tore-s) and (no-see-sep-tore-s).

Yes, they sound like members of the dinosaur family, but stick with me on this one. Can you name your five senses?

How did you do?

Here's the answers: Smell. Taste. Sight. Hearing. Touch.

Well done. What about your sixth sense? I bet you didn't know you have a sixth sense, did you? (And no I'm not talking about the movie). Your sixth sense is called "joint sense." Here's what I mean. Shut your eyes and hold your hand in front of you while doing the "peace" sign. Keep your arm there and count to ten. Go ahead. Give it a try. Did you do it?

Now, consider this: You could not smell or taste your fingers when they were in front of you (or at least I hope not). You could not see or hear your arm and fingers. And you didn't have to touch your arm using your other hand to know that it was extended, did you? And yet, I'm sure you were certain that you had your arm and hand in the right position. How is that possible? Through, your sixth sense, joint sense, that's how.

Joint sense is provided by a special set of nerves that tell your brain exactly what your joints are doing at all times. It's what allows your brain to "see" your joints so it knows how to control them. I bet you didn't know this, but most of the work of your brain involves coordinating and controlling your muscles and joints. Dr. Roger Sperry, 1981 Nobel Prize winner for brain research, found that "90 percent of the brain's energy output is relating the physical body to gravity." That's pretty impressive considering all of the other stuff the brain is responsible for doing.

The ins and outs of "joint sense" can get pretty technical, so let's try to keep it simple. When we break it down, you have two types of "joint sense" nerves.

1 You have nerves that tell your brain when your joints are moving in a good way. A "good way" is a way that doesn't damage the joints—when they stay within normal limits. This kind of movement keeps them healthy, and you want as much of this as possible. This is called *mechanoreception*, and these nerves are capable of detecting micrometers of change. That's really small. Like one millionth of a meter small. Think of a car "*mec*hanic" whose job it is to work with the structure and function of your car. In the same way, these nerves deal with the alignment (structure) and movement (function) of your joints (except they don't wear blue overalls). So that's mechanoreception.

2 Other nerves tell your brain when your joints are positioned and moving in a bad way. A "bad way" is a way that is outside of normal limits—and when it happens, your joints get damaged. This is called *nociception*, and you want as little of this as possible. Think of it as *"not good"* reception, and your brain is being told that everything is not okay. So that's nociception.

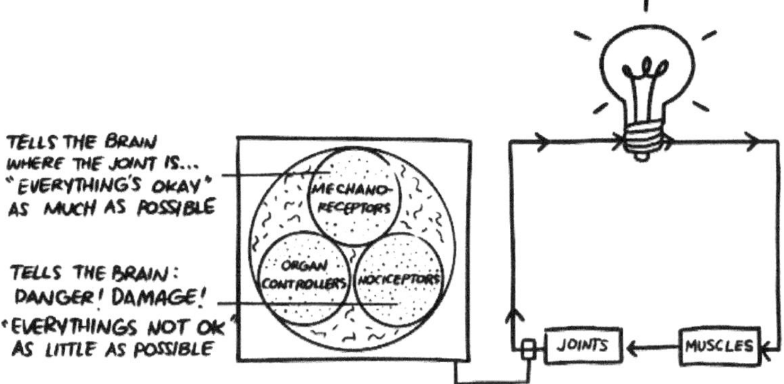

Remember what *mechanoreception* and *nociception* mean because you're going to see the words time and time again. This next part is important.

When your mechanoreceptors fire up, your brain knows that your joints are doing okay and it, in turn, responds appropriately. If, however, your nociceptors fire up, your brain knows that that the joints are in trouble, and it responds in a way, if left unchecked, that will eventually lead to pain. On top of that, nociception also can cause something called a "stress response," which is not good, either.

Pause a moment before reading any further. If the difference between the two categories of "joint sense" nerves isn't perfectly clear to you, please go back and re-read from the beginning of this chapter. If you don't get it, you won't fully appreciate how The Vicious Cycle or The Solution are important in becoming pain-free.

The Basics: Nerves resist sending messages.

A physical barrier/threshold keeps nerves from being too active, and it ensures that when nerves are not supposed to fire messages, they don't. This is like how the pain threshold ensures that when you're not supposed to feel pain, you don't. We don't want any old thing to cause a nerve to fire. It takes persistence. The *thing*—whether it be damage, hot, cold, vibration, touch, whatever—has to be big enough and happen often enough to cross the threshold. Only then will the nerve send off a message to the brain telling it what's happening—that's how nerves "resist." Really, this barrier is a way to keep our nerves in check, and it's to our advantage that we're pre-wired with this function because, if the nerves were allowed to fire off at their slightest whim, our world would fall into complete chaos. We'd be nervous wrecks. Once again, take a moment and study the graph below before moving on.

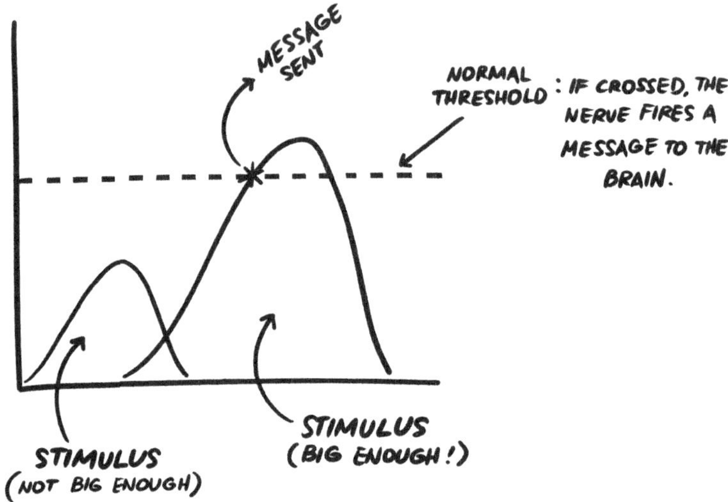

Some diseases disrupt the threshold and weaken resistance. Consider Parkinson's disease, for example. With this devastating ailment, the brain loses its ability to provide the chemicals necessary to resist the firing of nerves. And once the resistance is lost, muscles go haywire leading to shakiness, tremor, slowness, difficulty walking, and a whole host of other problems.

So the stronger your barrier, the stronger your resistance, the harder it is for the threshold to get crossed, and the more likely it is that the nerves won't be used when they're not supposed to be used. On the other hand, the weaker your barrier, the weaker your resistance, the easier it is for the threshold to be crossed, and the more likely it is that nerves will be used when they're not supposed to be used. This will be of great consequence in your pursuit of a pain-free life.

The Basics: Nerves can learn.

Nerves have a very special ability to learn. It's called "plasticity." Take learning how to play the piano, for instance. At first, it's difficult to get your fingers to move and hit the right keys. Ask any parent who has encouraged their child to take piano lessons—and then came to regret it. In the beginning, they hear a lot more ear-piercing music than ear-pleasing music. With practice, the fingers dance across the keyboard and the music becomes enjoyable. Watch a professional pianist play, and it's almost unreal how fast his fingers fly across the black and whites. It looks like the body is doing it automatically—because it is. Plasticity is found in the nerves, and is the ability to learn through repetition. The same principal is used in the martial arts, athletics, and singing. Everything you've ever learned, and have the potential to learn, is because of this ability. The constant use of nerves lowers their resistance, making them fire more readily. So for a piano virtuoso, playing becomes easier and easier the more he practices. That's plasticity.

It's why, as children, we are able to learn how to crawl, walk, and run. Whatever that *thing* you do is, plasticity allows that *thing* to be done easier the next time you do it. But what if that *thing* isn't being good at playing piano? What if that *thing* is bad? What if that *thing* is incorrect movement of your back and neck? What if that *thing* is poor posture? What if that *thing* is the nociceptors being repeatedly fired? What happens then?

Good questions, and you'll learn the answer in the next section. Look for the words "sensitization" and "neoneuralization."

The Basics: The two types of muscle.

You have two types of muscles in your body, and when they are in balance your back and neck are healthy and pain-free. They are:

1. Superficial, joint-moving muscles —The Movers
2. Deep, joint-stabilizing muscles—The Stabilizers

The "Movers" are designed to do just that—move you. These muscles generate power to propel you. Whether you're walking down the hall or sprinting through a field, the Movers do it. These muscles have names you are probably familiar with: deltoids, pecs, quads, biceps, etc. You may not have heard of some, like the trapezius and levator scapulae. The crucial thing to remember about these muscles is it's their nature to dominate, so they have to be kept in check. And that's where the "Stabilizers" come in.

The "Stabilizers" are designed to prevent the Movers from doing too much. They hold the joints together, protecting them. These muscles go by tongue-twisting names like multifidi, rotatares, gluteus medius, quadratus lumborum, and intertransversarii. You've probably never heard of them before, but believe me, they are important

As I mentioned earlier, the Stabilizers and the Movers have an intimate relationship. The Movers depend on the Stabilizers to anchor down the joints as they move us from Point A to Point B. Whether you are a professional body builder squatting four hundred pounds or an accountant squatting to pick up a piece a paper, these muscle groups have to work together in a coordinated manner. Your Movers move your joints so that you can live life—walk, jump, climb, sit down, bend over, etc. Your Stabilizers keep your Movers in check by anchoring down the joints, ensuring that the movement of your joints stays within healthy limits. When both muscle groups are equally strong and are coordinated with each other, they are considered "in balance." If the coordination is thrown off, the muscles become out-of-balance, and major problems enter your life.

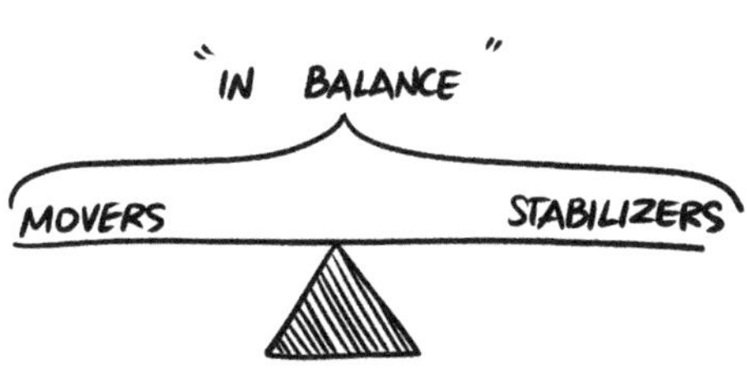

The Basics: Joints receive nourishment through a pumping process called "cyclic loading."

How well this "pump" functions depends on how well the joints move. This question may seem completely out-of-the blue, but play along with me. Why is your tongue one of the fastest healing tissues in your body? Here's a hint: it's why it's red.

The answer is blood. Your tongue possesses an incredible amount of tiny blood vessels that supply it with more than enough blood to keep it flushed with nutrients. This is what gives it that fast-healing ability.

Follow-up question: Why is cartilage one of the slowest healing tissues in your body? Hint: it's why it's yellowish gray.

Again, the answer is blood. But this time it's the lack thereof. You see, daily activities like bending and walking make it impossible for delicate blood vessels to survive inside the cartilage of the joints—there is too much stress and pressure. Because of this, for the most part, cartilage does not have a direct supply line of blood, and is therefore not chocked full of blood, hence its yellowish grey color. In order for cartilage to be healthy and pain-free, it has to get its nutrients through different means.

It accomplishes this through an amazing, self-healing mechanism that harnesses the unique characteristics of your joints to their own advantage: a pump.

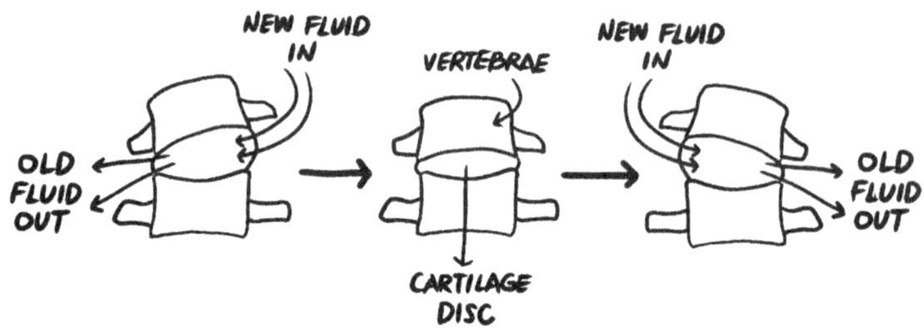

"THE PUMP" OF CYCLIC LOADING

Through a process called "cyclic loading," every movement you make does two things. It pumps new fluid and nutrients into the joint while simultaneously pumping out old fluid, and it stimulates new cartilage growth. The combination of these two processes is what keeps cartilage strong and resilient. Because this "cyclic-loading pump" is so efficient, joints should last about 110 years without premature deterioration and pain.

Every time you take a step, this pumping happens to your knee cartilage. Every time you bend over, this happens to the cartilage discs of your spine. As long as you are moving, you are repetitiously squeezing and stimulating your joint's cartilage (kind of like playing an accordion). Although your cartilage doesn't have a direct blood supply like the tongue to keep itself healthy, this ingenious pumping mechanism is more than enough.

By the way, it's important to note that all movements are not equally good for your joints. In the above examples you need to be loading your knee and lower back cartilage within healthy limits in order to reap the benefits of this pump.

A Quick Recap

You might be thinking "Okay, Doc, I understand this nerve-muscle-joint connection, but who cares? Why does this matter, really?"

When your joints move within healthy limits, the mechanoreceptors fire. Using this information your brain, in turn, tells your Stabilizers and Movers how to respond in a coordinated and balanced manner to keep the joints moving properly. This allows for optimal pumping so that your joints are preserved as close to pain-free as possible. In this collaborative way, your nerves, muscles, and joints work together to form one of the most important systems in your body: the aforementioned Neuromusculoskeletal System. Each component is essential to this cycle. When one element works well, it helps the others do the same.

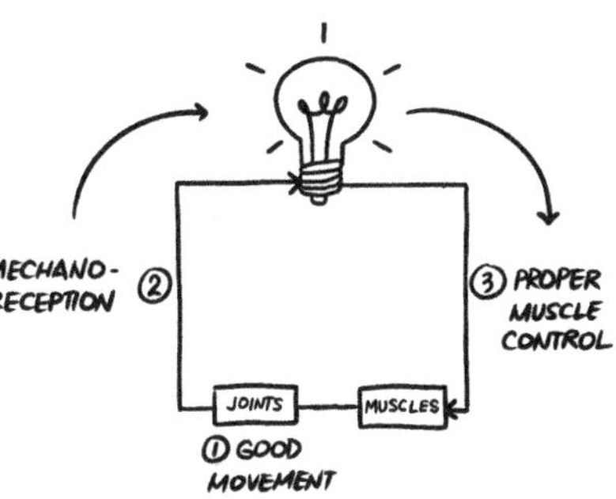

The Basics: Can an unhealthy spine make you sick?

Imagine an empty room. In the middle of that room sits a stationary bicycle. On the rear wheel of the bicycle is some type of contraption. Upon closer inspection you realize it's an electrical generator, and a power cord runs from it, along the floor, and up the wall where it connects to a light bulb. Now, imagine you're sitting on the bike and you begin to pedal. As you do, the light turns on.

When you stop, the light turns off, leaving you in darkness. You start again and the light turns on again. You pedal faster and the light gets brighter. After a while, you become fatigued, and you slow down. What do you notice about the light? It gets dimmer. Slower and slower you pedal until the light is barely a flicker. You stop and it turns off. Once again, you're left in darkness.

What you imagined here explains how your neuromusculoskeletal system impacts your health. The stationary bike represents your joints. The power cord represents your mechanoreceptors. And the light bulb represents your brain. Makes sense, doesn't it?

It is through the activity of the neuromusculoskeletal system that the brain is powered. In the same way that sunlight is essential for a flower to grow, movement is essential for your brain to be healthy. And the healthier your brain, the healthier every cell, tissue, and organ is in your body.

This is why walking thirty minutes a day has been proven to[1]:

- Prevent 47 percent of cognitive impairment
- Prevent 62 percent of Alzheimer's
- Prevent 52 percent of dementia
- Enhance learning by 12 times
- Decrease depression by 20 percent, including relapses
- Reduce the risk of breast cancer, pancreatic, lung, and colon cancer by 50 percent or more
- Prevent 50 percent of all stroke deaths
- Reduce congestive heart disease deaths by 63 percent
- Reduce hospital readmission for heart failure patients by 70 percent

And the list goes on and on.

It's not that exercise directly makes our hearts healthier, our immune systems stronger, and our brains keener. It's that exercise is movement, and movement activates mechanoreceptors that supply the brain with an essential nutrient—stimulation. Then the brain, in turn, makes our hearts healthier, immune systems stronger, and itself keener. It does this by releasing certain hormones that help keep every part of us well, including our internal organs. The details of this activity are outside the scope of this book, but—and trust me on this—this is basically how it works.

It's imperative to realize that not all joints have the same amount of influence on your brain's health, however. Compared to all of your other joints, your spine has by far the biggest impact on your brain's health and your body's wellbeing.

And it's not just any movement that causes good hormones to be released. Only good movement—the kind that stimulates mechanoreceptors and keeps the light bulb burning brightly—does that.

Again, Dr. Roger Sperry said that: "90 percent of the brain's stimulation and nutrition is generated from the movement of the spine."

So when the nerves, muscles, and joints of the spine are as healthy as possible, not only are you as pain-free as possible, but your whole body is healthier, too. This is why your spine matters, and why you should care for it. Now, let me be clear, you have to do other things to really increase your potential for optimal health. You know the drill: like eating good nutritious food, getting a good night's sleep, drinking plenty of water, etc. But still the fact remains that in our modern era, the spine is one of the most undervalued, underleveraged, and misunderstood components to a healthy, pain-free life. So yes, you do have a spine. Yes, it does impact your health. Yes, it does affect your life. And, yes, you do have to take care of it.

But what happens if you make a mistake?

- What happens if the neuromusculoskeletal system gets disrupted?
- What if the joints move incorrectly?
- What happens if the nociceptors, not the mechanoreceptors, fire?
- What if a nerve's resistance breaks down?
- What if the balance between the two muscle groups is thrown off?
- What if the nutrient pump shuts down?
- What happens if the light bulb begins to dim? What then?

The intimate connection between the nerves, muscles, and joints ends up *hurting* you instead of *helping* you—the light bulb goes dim and shuts off. And when this occurs, it is singlehandedly your greatest threat to getting pain-free. The cycle turns from doing "good" to doing "bad," and it is unforgiving, unrelenting, and it will be vicious.

Chapter 15

Summarizing Section 3

During a test; people look up for inspiration, down in desperation, and left and right for information.—Anonymous

We've covered quite a lot of information in this last section, so before moving on to the next, it's important that you've acquired the basic know-how to get the most out of The Vicious Cycle and The Solution. In order to do that, I'm going to test you, much like the test required to obtain a learner's permit for driving a car. In this case, you must answer 9 out 10 questions correctly to move on. If you do not meet this requirement, I encourage to go back and look up the answers. And if you pass, congratulations! You're another step closer to becoming pain-free.

Good luck!

1. The purpose of pain is:
    a. To make life uncomfortable
    b. Remind you that you're aging
    c. To serve as a warning against damage
    d. To give you something to talk about at your next family gathering

2. True or False: If you are in not currently in pain, it means there are absolutely no problems with your neck or back.
3. Immediately following damage to your body __________ occurs because it sets the groundwork for the next step in the healing process:
    a. Heat
    b. Pain
    c. Swelling
    d. Redness
    e. All of the above because they're all a part of infla-mmation
4. Mechanoreceptors detect:
    a. Cold
    b. Heat
    c. Moisture
    d. Joint position and movement
5. Nociceptors detect:
    a. Cold
    b. Damage
    c. Pressure
    d. "Bad" joint movement
    e. Both "b" and "d"
6. True or false: A nerve's "threshold" provides resistance so that when a nerve is not supposed to fire a message, it doesn't.
7. The ability of a nerve to "learn" is called
    a. Adaptability
    b. Plasticity
    c. Learning curve
    d. None of the above

8. The "Stabilizer" muscle group:
    a. Prevents the "Movers" from doing too much
    b. Holds joints together
    c. Protects joints
    d. All of the above
9. True or false: If the balance between the Movers and the Stabilizers is disrupted, the coordination between the two muscle groups *improves*.
10. Which of these is not a characteristic of "cyclic loading"?
    a. It supplies joints with nourishment
    b. Is highly dependent on how well the joints move
    c. Is needed because cartilage has a vast supply of blood vessels
    d. Keeps the joints healthy and pain-free

Answers:

1. C
2. False
3. E
4. D
5. E
6. True
7. B
8. D
9. False
10. C. Cyclic loading is need because cartilage has a poor supply of blood vessels.

SECTION 4

UNDERSTANDING THE PROBLEM: THE VICIOUS CYCLE

We cannot solve our problems with the same level of thinking that created them.—Albert Einstein, world renowned physicist

Chapter 16

The Buckling Point

It is unfortunate that so few appreciate from what small causes disease come.—Charles H. Mayo, M.D., founder of the Mayo Clinic

The first step down the Vicious Cycle's slippery slope is not dramatic. Quite the opposite. It's barely noticeable, and that's what makes it so sinister. This initial event is when a Buckling Point is created in the neck or back. A Buckling Point is the moment in time when a joint is pushed outside of its normal limits, causing nociceptors to fire.

A Buckling Point can be created two ways in your back and neck. The first way is when *Something Bad Happens To You*—when an outside force impacts your body and causes damage. Examples of this include a slip, fall, car accident, being tackled, etc. It's the outside force's fault that a Buckling Point was created.

The second and far more common way is when *You Do Something Wrong.* You control how you move and bend your spine, and when you use it incorrectly, you can force your spinal joints outside of their normal healthy limits. This means it's your fault that a Buckling Point was created.

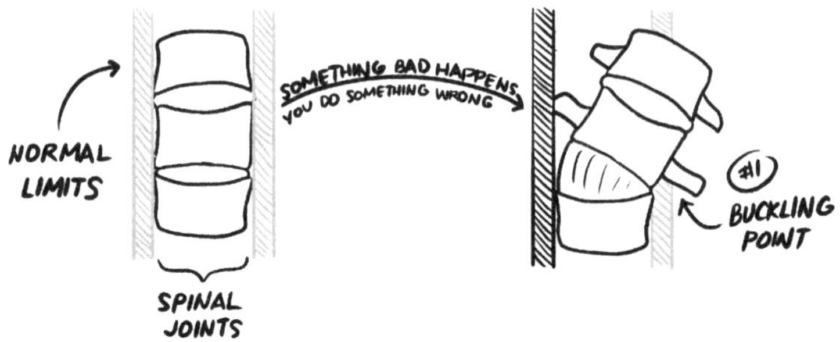

Now, once this happens and nociceptors send the first signals racing toward the brain, the message travels along the length of the nerve and to your spinal cord where a very peculiar reaction occurs: a muscle reflex which causes your Movers to contract and your Stabilizers to relax.

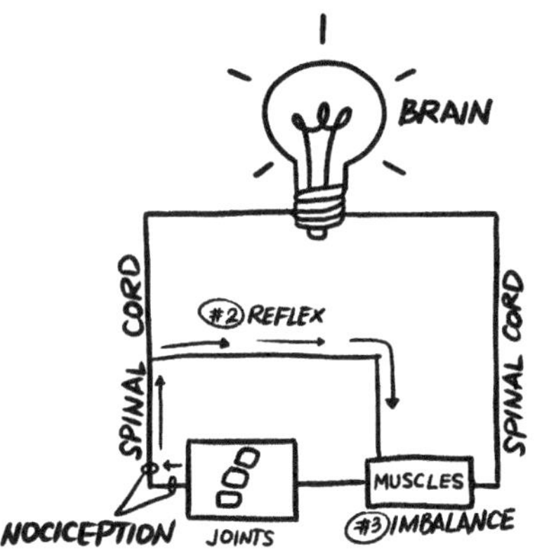

In fact, it's the same reflex that happens when a doctor hits your kneecap with that reflex hammer…and your leg jumps. It jumps because when the kneecap's tendon is quickly stretched, the leg Mover called your quadriceps—the front leg muscle that makes up your thigh—instantly and fully contracts, and at the same time, the Stabilizers of your knee become momentarily flaccid/limp.

When nociceptors fire because of a Buckling Point, this reflex is sparked, but on a much smaller scale, causing the delicate balance between the two muscle groups to get thrown off. Instead of the Movers going all-out and fully contracting, they are "facilitated," which means that for a moment it simply gets easier for them to contract. In the same instance the Stabilizers, instead of going flaccid, are "inhibited," which means it gets harder for them to contract.

At this point your body goes one of two ways. Option "A" is that the Buckling Point "recovers," meaning that the nociceptors have stopped firing, and normal muscle balance has been restored. This brings the joint back to within normal limits. Although we are, for the most part, completely unaware of it, Buckling Point recovery happens thousands of times in a day.

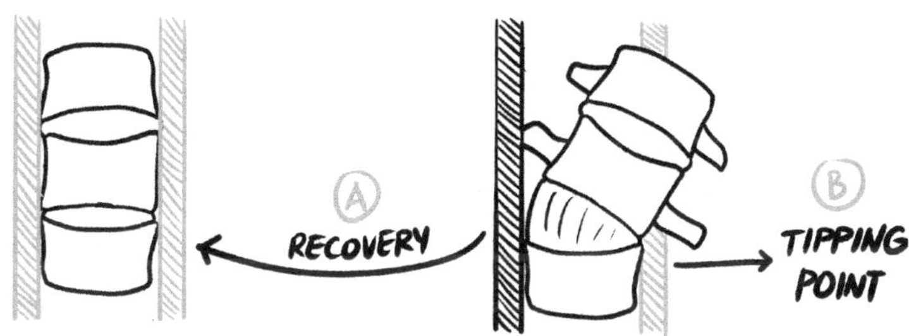

Option "B" is that the muscle balance does not get restored, and the Buckling Point does not recover, which forces that part of your spine into the next phase of the Vicious Cycle. What determines whether or not your joints recover? Here are a few factors:

1 How bad was the outside force? As long as it wasn't too big or traumatic, you'll be okay.
2 How did the outside force happen? Compressive injuries

(like squatting too much weight at the gym) or twisting injuries (like shoveling snow), are more complex and therefore less likely to recover on their own.

3 How long have you been doing something wrong? Let's say you've recently started a new job that requires you to sit. Unless you're careful, you'll invariably end up creating Buckling Points in your neck. You may be okay for the first few weeks, but if you've been at this seated job for years, you're going to have a problem.

4 How well do you eat? If you're deficient in key nutrients, you're less likely to bounce back. We'll address this issue more thoroughly in the last chapter.

5 Do you smoke? Nicotine weakens cartilage, making it harder to recover.

6 How stressed are you? The more stress you're under, the more likely you'll head further down the Vicious Cycle.

7 How old are you? The older you are, the harder it is for your body to turn around.

The list goes on and on, but you get the point. It's never only one thing that determines whether or not your joints recover from a Buckling Point. A whole host of factor contribute. What's important to understand is that eventually Something Bad *will* Happen or You *will* Do Something Wrong which will create a Buckling Point that *cannot* recover. And when that moment occurs, you've hit a Tipping Point.

Summary

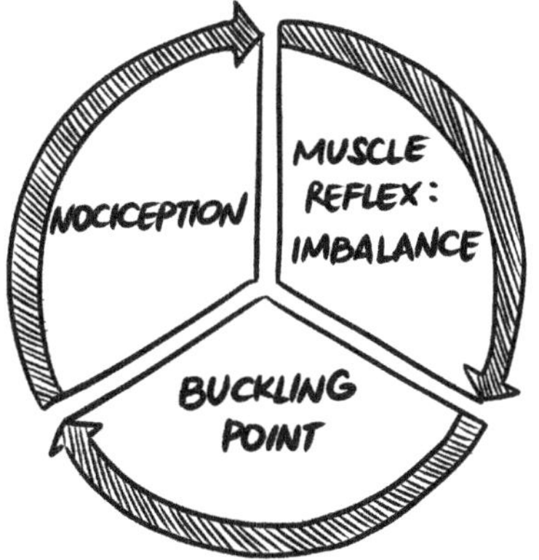

Chapter 17

The Tipping Point: Dysfunction

It is reasonable to suggest that the great majority of individuals suffer from asymptomatic joint dysfunction before spinal tissue injury generates pain.—James Chestnut, B.Ed., M.Sc., D.C., C.C.W.P., author of "The Wellness and Prevention Paradigm"

What happens next ultimately becomes the driving force behind the entire Vicious Cycle—it is the engine that moves the car. The tricky bit is that it occurs without a single symptom leaving many people unaware that their spine has started down a dangerous path. My hope is that you won't be part of that group. For reaffirmation, at the end of this section, I have included a "self-test" you should take which will determine whether or not this is happening to you. The results might be surprising.

The last section left off with nociceptors initiating a reflex that forced an imbalance between the Movers and the Stabilizers. Remember, these muscles move the joints, and to do so properly, they have to be balanced. When a Buckling Point occurs, and the muscles become imbalanced, their actions become uncoordinated, which results in the joint not moving properly. Instead of gliding smoothly, the joint moves erratically. If the reflex doesn't cease and muscle balance restored, the joint will stay moving like this, and will be officially designated as "dysfunctional." (What nerves detect this type of "bad" movement? Nociceptors.) After all this, nociceptors then begin firing repeatedly, and the once momentary reflex is now the standard operating procedure. This is when the Tipping Point has been crossed, and your back and neck have officially entered into the Vicious Cycle.

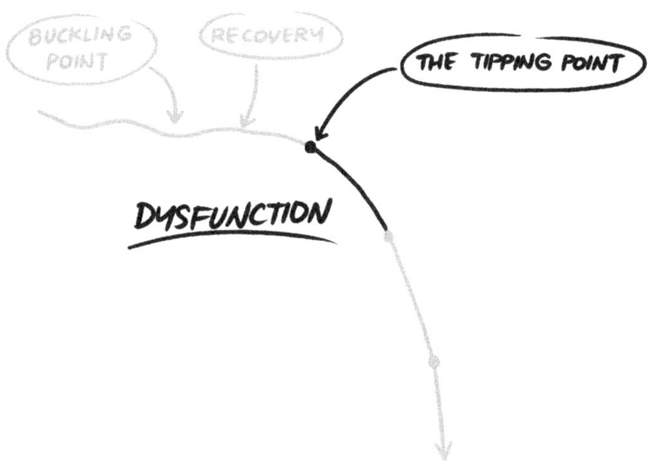

You see, before the Tipping Point you had to be hit by something, or you had to keep making mistakes in order to fire the nociceptors. But now, they fire whenever that dysfunctional joint moves (which will be every time you move your spine). After this point has been crossed, your back and neck are set on a course to develop problems and eventual pain. This is another paragraph worth rereading. The clear, uncompromising and downright depressing message: once you've reached the Tipping Point, any movement is another step closer to pain.

How lovely.

Worsening Dysfunction: The Muscles

Because the Movers have become facilitated, it's easy for them to contract and become overactive. From this, eventually, they tighten. Because of inhibition, it gets increasingly difficult for the Stabilizers to contract, so they tend to be underused and grow weaker. This causes the imbalance and incoordination between the two muscle groups to worsen.

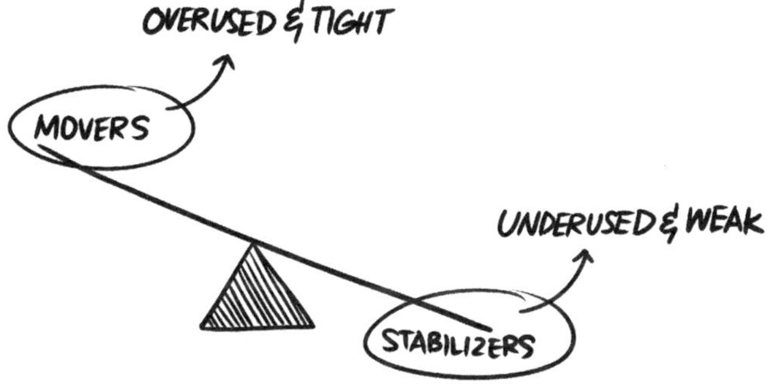

Worsening Dysfunction: The Joints

The growing severity of muscle imbalance and incoordination turns the joint's erratic movement into lack-of-movement. Losing mobility is bad because it structurally weakens joints. Remember, your joints depend on motion to "pump" nutrients into the cartilage and bone. Lack of mobility turns off the pump that flushes the joints with nutrients, thus it starves the cartilage and bone, weakening them.

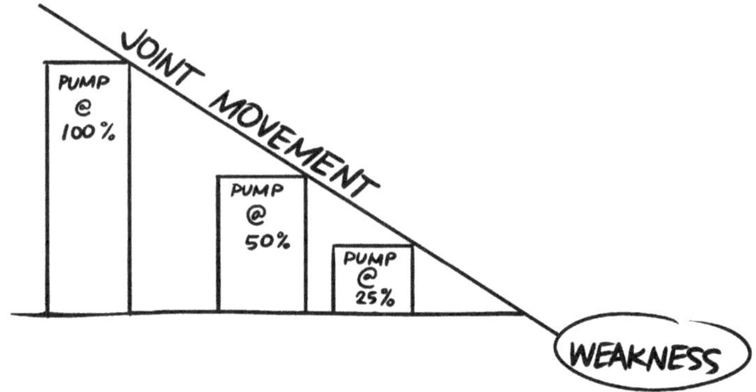

Worsening Dysfunction: The Big Wheel Keeps On Turning

- As the joints begin to weaken, do you think their mobility gets better or worse? *Worse.*
- With worsening mobility, do the nociceptors fire less or more? *More.*
- Does this put less or more stress on the muscles? *More.*
- What happens to their imbalance and incoordination? *It gets worse.*
- What does that do to the joint's mobility? *Gets even worse, making the joints even weaker.*

As long as the three elements—the nerves, muscles, and joints—are dysfunctional, the momentum of the Vicious Cycle continues to build.

It's important to note that although the joints aren't moving the way they should be moving, there isn't any damage yet. Here's a quote from the research:

> "Initially, there is abnormal motion of the spinal segment and pathological signs of degeneration are minimal; this stage being termed 'spinal dysfunction.'"[2]

There is an important concept in those words. They describe a "stage" where the back and neck have "abnormal motion" *before* "degeneration" occurs. They're saying that Dysfunction precedes Destruction, and it's not until something gets damaged that there is the potential for pain. Not only is this "dysfunctional" phase without symptoms, but it is also without damage—which is what makes it tricky to detect. Unfortunately, because of this many people are walking around completely oblivious that this is happening to their neck and back. Or worse, they know, but don't care because it's not causing pain...yet.

Which is complete lunacy.

Do we think plaque buildup on teeth is okay because it hasn't yet rotted out the tooth? Do we think a little bit of mold in a new house is no big deal because it's not out-of-control yet? Do we think elevated blood sugar levels aren't important because they haven't yet caused insulin resistance—a telltale sign of Type II diabetes?

Of course not. Everyone knows if a small problem isn't fixed, it only gets worse. Well, that's the Dysfunctional Phase in the Vicious Cycle—if you take care of this small weed now, it won't grow out of control.

If you can get the nociceptors to cease firing, the muscles will recover, and the Dysfunctional Phase will stop because the nerves, muscles, and joints still have the potential to return back to normal. In order to do so, *dys*-function must turn into function. For that to happen, the treatment must address all three elements equally and completely. This is why the standard approach to back and neck pain is such a complete failure—it simply doesn't do that. Most treatment available today allows the three elements to continue to feed off each other. Lucky for you, The Solution addresses all three elements thoroughly. You're almost there.

If the spinal dysfunction isn't caught and corrected, it will continue to worsen until the back and neck enter the next phase of the Vicious Cycle: The Destruction Phase.

Summary

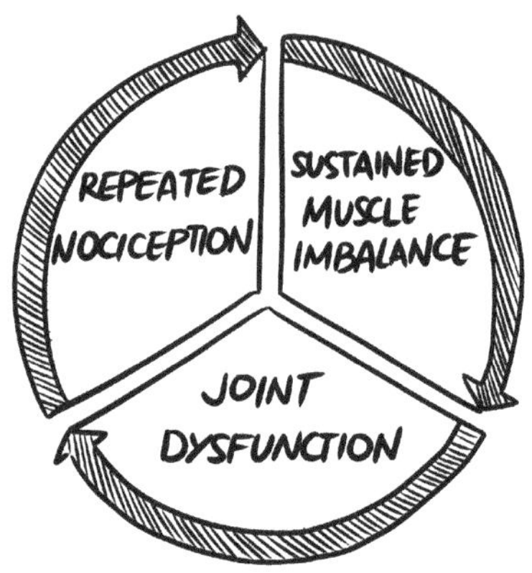

Self-Test

As you sit there reading this book, there's a good chance your back and neck is in a dysfunctional state right now. Curious? There's a simple way to determine if the base of your neck and mid-back have entered into this phase. I'll explain the test. Then when I say "go," give it a try. First, put the book down and let your arms rest loosely at your sides. Then, take a very, very deep breath in, as deep as you can manage. Ready? Go.

Okay, relax. Don't worry, no one is watching.

Now do it again. But this time pay attention to what your shoulders are doing.

Do they stay at one level? Do they rise up? Do they depress? Got it? Ready? Set. Go.

Here's how to interpret the test. If your shoulders elevated *at all*, you failed and your upper back and neck muscles are dysfunctional. If your neck and mid back Stabilizers were balanced and coordinated, your shoulders would not elevate. Instead, your belly would expand (called diaphragmatic breathing) and your shoulders would depress.

If you didn't pass, it could very well mean that your neck and mid back are currently dysfunctional. You've been warned!

Chapter 18

The Breaking Point: Destruction

Why did one straw break the camel's back? Here's the answer: the million other straws beneath it.—Mos Def

The saying "The straw that broke the camel's back" originates from ancient Egypt when camels were used to transport straw over long distances. It was well known that a camel could carry a certain amount of weight without any problems, but at a certain point, the camel's spine couldn't sustain any more weight. If that point was crossed, even by a single straw, the camel's back would break.

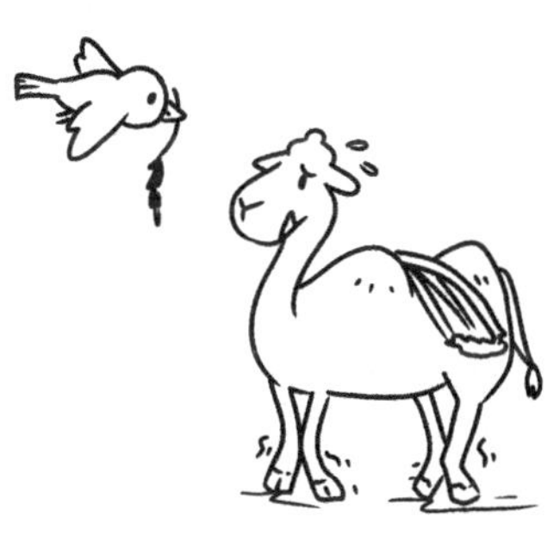

Get this. In the Dysfunctional Phase, this is exactly what your back and neck have been going through. Your nerves, muscles, and joints have had an increasing amount of stress put on them making it only a matter of time before they hit the Breaking Point—when Dysfunction turns into Destruction.

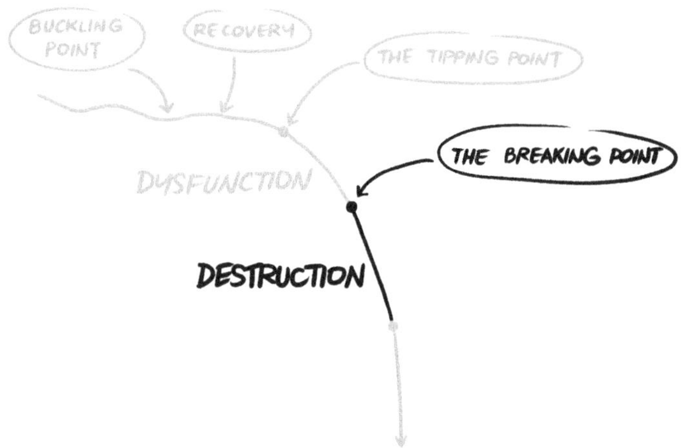

During this next phase, the slope of the Vicious Cycle gets much steeper. Your back and neck begin breaking down, which moves you away from being pain-free and healthy and closer to pain and sickness.

Destruction: The Nerves—Nociceptors

If you remember, nerves have a natural resistance that serves as a barrier against them firing too easily. During the Dysfunctional Phase that barrier remained untouched, but during the phase of Destruction, that wall comes tumbling down.

Here's how it happens.

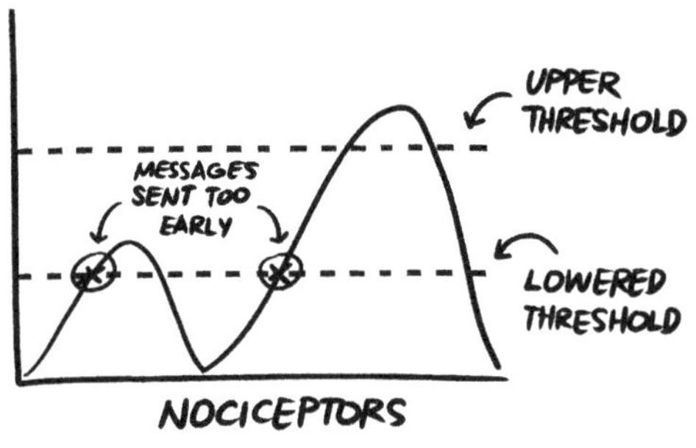

Prolonged, involuntary joint dysfunction forces nociceptors to fire over and over again, wearing down their resistance and lowering their threshold.

This means that it takes less stimulus to cause them to fire. In fact, the nociceptors become so "on edge" and "wound up" that they overreact at the slightest provocation. It can even get to the point where normal and healthy movements cause them to fire. This nerve-disease process has a name, and it's one you've seen before: sensitization (mentioned in the first pain myth).

If pain sets in while sensitization is present, it can make for a real mess. Ask any chronic pain sufferer. Activities that used to be done without thinking—like getting dressed in the morning—now cause the pain sufferer to move more warily.

Sensitization not only makes it easier for nociceptors to fire, but it is also a vehicle in which the Vicious Cycle spreads to other areas by corrupting adjacent nerves. Unless stopped, sensitization will infect the nerve down to its root: the spinal cord. This is disastrous because all nerves connect to the spinal cord, so once there, sensitization spreads like wildfire. Nerves that were functioning normally, three, four, or five segments away from the initial Dysfunctional Joint, now turn into sensitized, nociceptive zombies.

And, of course, *where nociception goes, dysfunction follows, and where dysfunction goes, destruction is soon to come.*

Note here that more nociception does not necessarily mean more pain. It certainly can, but it doesn't have too. In fact, believe it or not, everything described so far can still occur without any symptoms or pain. We only consciously comprehend a tiny fraction of what is happening with our bodies. When I say tiny, I mean .0000000000016 percent. Don't let yourself be fooled into thinking you would know if this was happening to your back and neck. I've heard dozens of patients, hunched over in pain, say things like, "This just came out of nowhere." The truth is that back problems never come from out of nowhere. They always come from somewhere, and that somewhere is usually nociception and the Vicious Cycle.

Destruction: The Nerves—Mechanoreceptors

While nociceptors are being sensitized, the exact opposite is happening to the mechanoreceptors. Their threshold increases, building resistance, making it more difficult for them to fire.

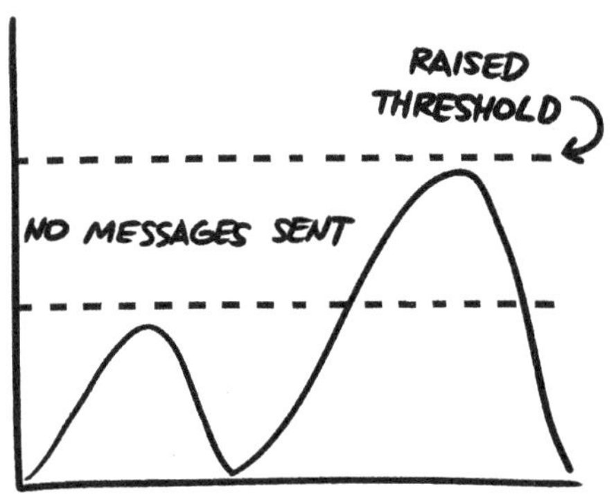

This forces the mechanoreceptors to be less active, and in the end this lack of use causes their pathways to deteriorate—like an old, underused, and under-cared-for road. It becomes difficult for them to do their job of feeding the brain information about what the joints are doing. Since the brain depends on mechanoreceptors to "see" the joints and control them, this lack of signaling causes the brain to become essentially "blind" to those joints. This allows for more severe muscle and joint dysfunction.

This "blindness" can get so bad that without help, you won't be able to move your body the way you're supposed to. I see people in this stage nearly every day in my clinic. I'll ask a patient to perform a very simple move with his neck or lower back, one that most six-year-olds can perform easily, but the man won't be able to do it. I'll explain it again, walking him through the steps. He'll try again and fail. At this point, I'll have to demonstrate the move so he can see how to do it. I'll have him try it again, and he may fail again. When it gets to this point, I'll have to grasp him and move his neck or back for him so he can feel it. It may take a few sessions of this type of one-on-one attention, but after a while he'll start to do it right. You see, it's because his brain lacks mechanoreception that he lost the ability to move his neck or back the way he's supposed to, and the only way to change this is to turn the mechanoreceptors back on. That's *exactly* what The Solution does.

Destruction: The Muscles—The Stabilizers

First, the Stabilizers begin to atrophy (a medical word for "to waste away"). The reflex that made it more difficult for the Stabilizers to contract worsens and causes them to "shut off" like a light switch. Eventually, they weaken and start withering away like an unwatered lawn in the heat of summer.

This has profound implications for the healing process. In the Dysfunctional Phase, the Stabilizers simply need to be re-awakened in order to restore their normal function and eliminate pain, but in the Destruction Phase, they have to be completely rebuilt—a much more involved process.

Destruction: The Muscles—The Movers

While this is happening to the Stabilizers, the Movers begin to go through their own type of destruction. During the Dysfunctional Phase, the nociceptors forced the Movers to become overactive. When they should be resting, they're working, and when they're supposed to be working, they overdo it. At first the Movers can handle this extra activity and stress, but it's not long before they hit their Breaking Point and begin to micro-tear.

Unless you're well versed in the world of physical medicine, you've probably never heard of a micro-tear. Let me explain.

A muscle is made of millions of tiny, individual muscle fibers—much like how a rope is made of smaller fibers. If that rope is suddenly put under a lot of tension, it will completely tear. If that happens to a muscle, it's called a rupture, which can occur, for instance, by falling on an outstretched arm. If a rope has stress or tension that's quite small at the beginning, but slowly increases, it won't suddenly fail, but rather its individual fibers will start to break one-by-one on its way to giving out. That's micro-tearing.

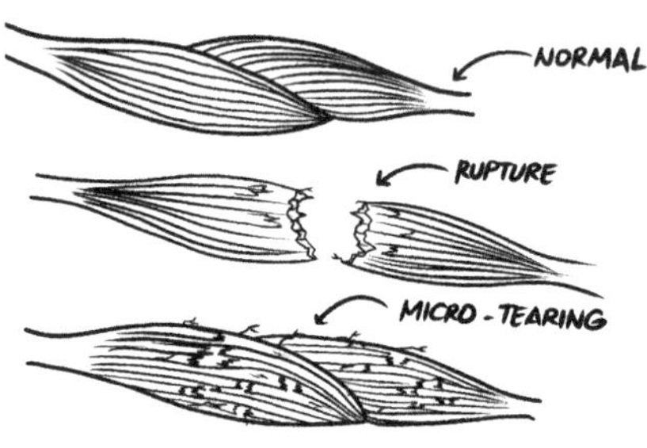

With atrophying Stabilizers and micro-tearing Movers making the muscle imbalance and incoordination more profound, destruction to the joints is soon to follow.

Destruction: The Joints

At this point, because of erratic movement and overall lack of joint mobility, the flushing of nutrients into the joint has basically stopped. Firstly, this causes a buildup of inflammatory metabolic "waste" that begins to eat away at the joint from the inside out like acid. Secondly, lack of pumping severely starves the cartilage and bone, literally killing the cells. This combination results in destruction. Here's how:

- **Synovial fluid** (the oil in between the joints): It gets used up faster than it can be replaced, resulting in a liquid that's too watery to protect and lubricate. This leaves the cartilage exposed to too much friction. This is like what would happen to your car's engine if you were to put in the wrong kind of motor oil.

- **Articular cartilage** (the thin layer of cartilage that cover the ends of bones): The loss of synovial fluid, and increase in friction, causes this cartilage to wear thin. The resulting lack-of-cushion puts increased stress on the underlying bone.
- **Bone** (i.e., vertebrae): After the protective cartilage has worn away, the bone begins to feel the burn of friction, ultimately causing damage and bone death.
- **Intervertebral discs:** As the cells that form its cartilage begin to die off, the layers of the disc begin to separate, tear, and collapse like an old, run-down building. This structural damage robs the disc's ability to handle stress and the body's weight. Result: much faster degradation. It's during this phase that the disc is likely to herniate, "slip," or bulge.

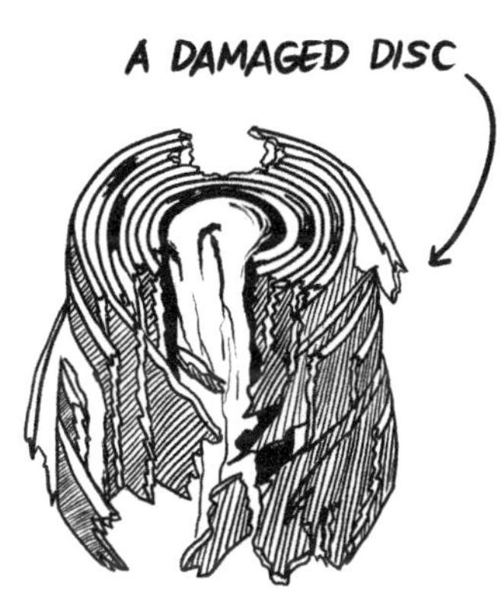

As all of this is going on, what do you think is happening to the joint's alignment and mobility?

It gets much worse. Sooner rather than later, the dysfunction and destruction of one joint begins to spread, affecting entire regions of the spine. No longer is it only one spot in the neck that is problematic, now it's the whole neck. This brings about even more nociception and more destruction in the nerves, muscles, and joints allowing the Vicious Cycle to build more momentum until one defining moment occurs—The Point of No Return.

Summary

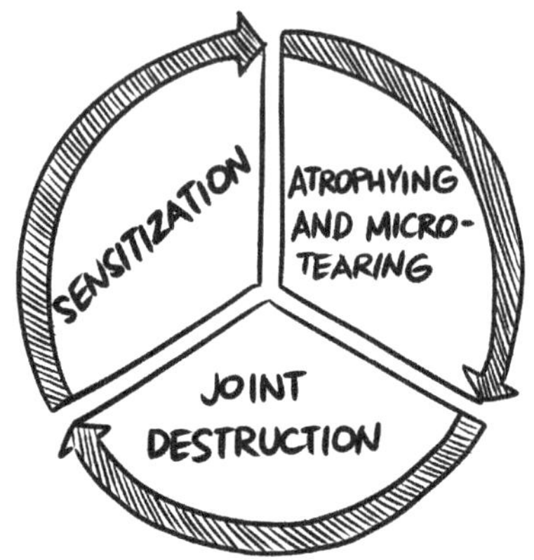

Chapter 19

The Point of No Return: Pathological Protection

...it is useful to consider degeneration not as an inevitable process, but as one that is initiated by some mechanical or nutritional insult and superimposed on normal aging.—Michael A. Adams, BSc, PhD

Your brain thinks your back and neck are important. I hope you're starting to think so, too. When dysfunction has occurred in the spine, it is a dangerous situation—your nerves and spinal cord, essential components of staying alive, are at risk. When destruction sets in, the downward slope of the Vicious Cycle turns into a cliff, and the body enters into a free-fall of an ever-worsening condition. If this trend isn't stopped, there comes a point when the back and neck have deteriorated so much that your brain takes matters into its own hands.

When the Point of No Return is crossed, your brain understands that your spine needs attention, and realizes that you're either unwilling or unable help it. This is an emergency, and the brain issues a "code red" alert, moving the back and neck into a phase of

Pathological Protection—when the nerves, muscles, and joints start to protect themselves. It's a particularly vicious step because these actions cannot be taken back. Once you hit this point in the Vicious Cycle, it's impossible to get your spine all the way back to being completely normal and healthy. That's the bad news. The good news is that this doesn't mean there is no hope for you. Hitting The Point of No Return does not mean you cannot live a life mostly free of pain. But it *does* means you have a lot of work ahead of you.

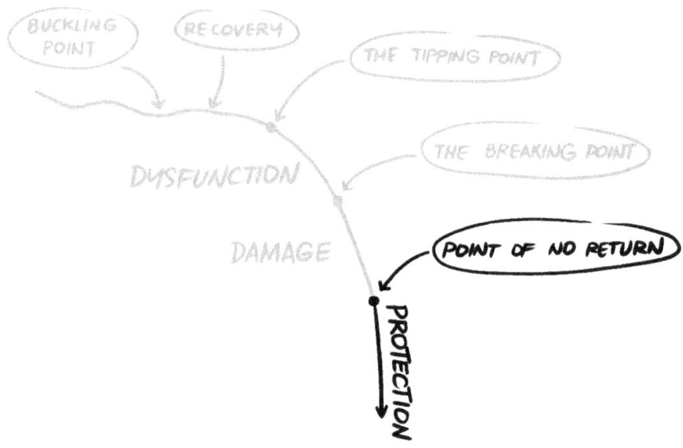

Pathological Protection: The Nerves

This is when we can actually start to feel the sensitization that the nerves have been going through. First, the back and neck develop "hyperalgesia" (definition: hyper = over, algesia = pain) which refers to an abnormally intense pain response induced by a *painful* stimulus. Example: when your grandson jumps on your back, you're sore for the next three weeks. You knew it would hurt, but you didn't think it would hurt that bad and for that long.

After that, the back and neck develop "allodynia," which refers to pain that occurs in response to *harmless* stimuli. This is when something shouldn't hurt, but does. In my practice, I have firsthand experience with these phenomena. I examine patients, and no matter where I touch their back, they nearly jump off the exam table in pain. I have patients tell me that simply brushing up against a wall or the slightest change in weather causes pain. (Keep in mind that both hyperalgesia and allodynia are driven by sensitization, which develops from constant nociceptive firing due to abnormal joint movement.)

Not only do the nerves become more sensitive to pain, but new nerves can grow into areas of damage, like disc and muscle. The process of new nerve growth in dysfunctional and damaged tissue is called "neoneuralization" (neo = new, neural = nerve, ization = "the process of"). When you combine this with allodynia, it creates a really sticky mess for people. Think about it. At this point, your body is creating more nerves that are able to feel more pain.

Those last three paragraphs are important, so take some time, and read them again.

It's true. Nerves become more sensitive to pain, and your body reacts by growing more nerves to stimulate more pain. What's up with that? Isn't that a bit masochistic? Why do the nerves start to feel more pain? Remember the purpose of pain? It's a warning—and it's for your protection. The nervous system starts to go down this path because if you do *something* that hurts, chances are you won't do that *something* again. That's how the nerves start to protect your back and neck.

I'm reminded of a patient who sought my care following a second failed spinal surgery. When she came in, she couldn't stand for longer than five minutes without severe low-back pain. A side bend made her yelp in pain. The act of getting on the exam table and lying on her stomach brought her to tears. When I started to feel her back, assessing her muscle tone, she yelled in pain.

She was a mess.

Now this woman was one of the sweetest people I've ever met, and it broke my heart to see her in so much pain. I point this out because The Vicious Cycle doesn't care who you are. It doesn't care if you're rich or poor; overweight or in good shape; famous or not well-known; young or old; or African American, Caucasian, Hispanic, or Asian. If a Buckling Point is created in your spine, this is what happens. Once the Tipping Point is crossed, it has to be thoroughly addressed, otherwise it gets worse. If it crosses the Point of No Return, permanent changes have occurred and it is considerably harder to become pain-free.

Be careful!

Pathological Protection: The Muscles

Although the muscles are atrophied and micro-tearing, they are still forced to do their job day in and day out. When you drive, for instance, you still have to turn your head to check your blind spot. You still have to carry the groceries in from the car. You still have to bend over to pick up the dirty clothes that you, or more likely your kids, dropped on the floor. This never-ending use of broken-down muscle tissue interferes with its healing process. The atrophied muscles are trying to rebuild, and the micro-tears are trying to repair, but they can't because the Vicious Cycle has brought them so far away from the environment they need for healing they have to take action to protect themselves.

In an optimal environment, muscle heals muscle. In a suboptimal environment, scar tissue heals muscle.

When damaged muscles are caught in the Vicious Cycle, and they attempt to heal, scar tissue is laid down instead of new muscle fibers.

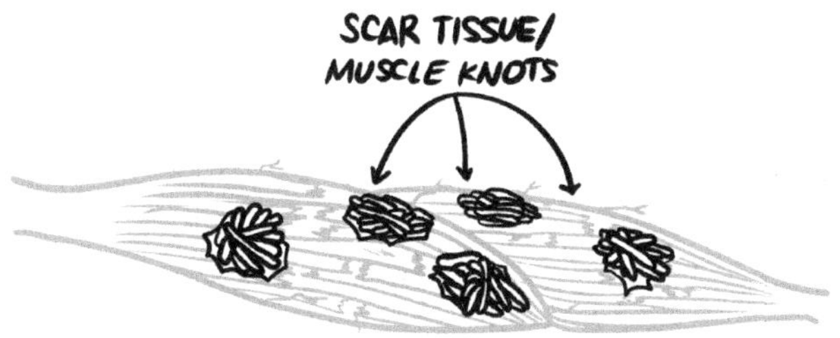

Scar tissue is non-flexible, short, and is altogether different from normal muscle tissue—much like how a scar on the skin is different than the skin itself.

You might ask, "How does scar tissue protect me?" Well, scar tissue is actually tougher than muscle tissue. That's why it's laid down. It's the body's way to protect the muscles from further tearing.

Unfortunately, there are many disadvantages to scar tissue.

1 Scar tissue doesn't look like muscle. Muscle is nice, smooth, and organized. Scar tissue, on the other hand, is a gnarled entanglement of dead muscle fibers, cartilage, and nerves.
2 Scar tissue causes more pain. Unlike scar tissue found in skin, which has less pain-sensitive nerves, scar tissue in muscle has more pain-sensitive nerves, making it a possible source, all by itself, of significant pain. Not good news for pain sufferers.
3 Scar tissue spreads. It tethers to surrounding muscles, causing otherwise normal muscles to become dysfunctional, and continues to throw off your muscle balance.
4 Scar tissue causes less mobility. Lack of mobility leads to

> loss of function. Loss of function results in that tissue, whether it's neck, back, shoulder, or knee, getting weaker and eventually re-aggravated—more often than not—by normal, everyday use.

While this may seem new to you, you've actually known about muscle scar tissue for quite some time, but by a different name: muscle knots. Scar tissue is what causes muscles to "knot up." In fact, go ahead and feel the knots at the base of your neck, by your shoulders. Think those are normal? Harmless? There for no reason? Ha! What you're feeling is overworked, under-rested, out-of-balance, scar-tissue-ridden muscles. Since we're on the topic, muscles do not simply develop "knots" out of the blue. People often say this, and you've probably said it yourself: "I have knots in my shoulders." "I have knots in my low back." And so on. What's actually happening is that scar tissue is tethering to the surrounding muscle, causing it to knot up.

I hope you understand why it makes me shudder when people nonchalantly say, "I always have knots there." They don't know that *so much has had to go wrong* in order for those "knots" to form.

Pathological Protection: The Joints

Up to this point, the weakened cartilage and bone have been getting damaged because they have been forced to keep you moving even though they don't have the ability to withstand the stress that comes with it. In response to this, changes occur within the cartilage and bone that stop the joint from being able to move because if the joint can't move, then movement can't hurt the joint. That makes sense, doesn't it? The only problem is that your level of activity is determined by your level of mobility, so if your joints move less, you move less, and if you move less, you do less.

Here are some of the changes that take place:

The intervertebral disc: as it breaks down, it goes from being soft and squishy to tough and inflexible. It goes from basically being a shock-absorbing water balloon to a rough leathery sack.

The bone (i.e., vertebrae): the parts that were under friction in the last phase now react by laying down new, thicker bone—kind of like scar tissue to muscle. Trouble is, the body doesn't lay down just enough to replace what was lost. Not a chance. The body adds layer upon layer of bone, causing the once nicely square vertebrae to develop jagged, gargoyle-looking bone spurs.

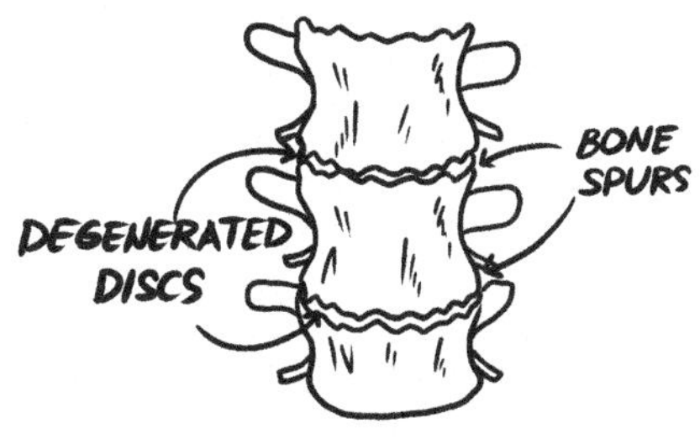

Not only that, but this outgrowing of bone can lead to the narrowing of the little holes through which the spinal nerves exit, causing a condition called *foraminal stenosis.* It can get so severe that the spinal canal—which houses the spinal cord—will start to narrow—a condition called *spinal stenosis.*

Why does the body do this? How does a bone spur protect your spine? Bone spurs, in fact, do two things: first, they stabilize the joint, and second, they increase the surface area available to the disc, thereby making it more resilient and stable. This is good until you realize what you're sacrificing—once again, mobility, and your ability to do what you want.

I hope you now understand why I almost fall off my chair when a patient casually mentions she's been told she has arthritis and some bone spurring, and there's really nothing that can be done. Remember, "It's normal," and "simply a part of aging," Right? WRONG! It has very little to do with "aging," and nearly everything to do with how deep into the Vicious Cycle you've traveled.

Keep this in mind. If you are ever shown an X-ray of your spine, and the doctor points at the image and says, "That's arthritis," or "That's degenerative joint disease," or "That's a bone spur," immediately look at the other joints and see if *all* of them have the *exact same amount* of arthritis, degeneration, or spurring. Chances are you'll see a joint that looks fine, like there's nothing wrong with it. If that's the case, do yourself a huge favor and ask the doctor, "Why is that area more broken down than the other area?" If he blows off your question with an answer like "aging," or "that's how it goes," or if they don't give you a clear answer that makes sense to you based on what you now understand of the Vicious Cycle, consider getting a second opinion.

If the doctor can't explain the difference to you, they don't have the right kind of knowledge to get you better.

The Bottomless Pit

Ignorance is not bliss. What you don't know about your body will hurt you.This is the reason why this part of the Vicious Cycle is called the "Point of No Return"—once you've gone this far, you can't make it all the way back. The brain has been forced to take command and, unfortunately, that means permanent changes. Once a bone spur is formed, it's there to stay. Once a certain amount of scar tissue has developed, it cannot be totally extricated. Once the nerves are so sensitized that you feel pain from by normal touch, they can't be totally desensitized. All of these things rob you of your mobility, activity level, and quality of life, and will lead you further and further down the Vicious Cycle and eventually into more and more pain.

The good news is that by applying The Solution, you will be able to show your brain that not only do you care, but you know how to care for your spine. This is the first and most important step to break the Vicious Cycle and rid yourself of pain once and for all.

Summary

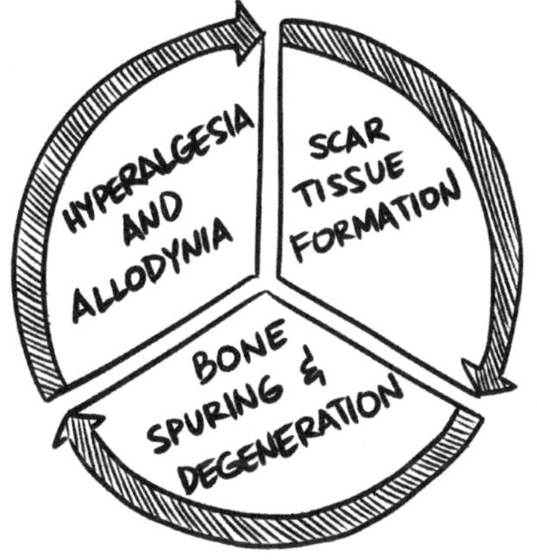

Chapter 20

The Final Point: Beyond the Vicious Cycle

It is the job of the spine to keep the brain alert. The moment the spine collapses, the brain collapses.—B.K.S. Iyengar, yoga master

We know that nociceptors send stress signals to the spinal cord, which then causes a reflex that leads to loss of balance and coordination in muscles, thus driving us further into the Vicious Cycle. But, those stress signals don't stop there. Their next destination is your brain, and from there, potentially, to every cell in your body.

Once the stress signal hits the spinal cord, it shoots up to the brain via the "spino-thalamo-cortico-pituitario-tract"—a fancy string of words that describe the pathways a nociceptor takes to the brain. You see, increased nociception can cause your brain to release "stress hormones," which are responsible for virtually every symptom of stress: increased heart rate, elevated blood pressure, increased feelings of stress, fear, anxiety, and depression. They're also responsible for symptoms you may not be aware of: insulin resistance, elevated blood sugar levels, a change in blood cholesterol profile, diminished immune system function, bone loss, and sensitivity to pain.

As the Vicious Cycle progresses, and the increasing amount of nociceptive stress signals continue to bombard the brain and more stress hormones are released, as Dr. James Chestnut notes:

> "Increased release of stress hormones drives the physiology of the body toward a state of alarm and adaption, and, if these levels remain elevated, can result in fatigue, illness, and early death."[5]

You want the least possible amount of stress hormones in your body at all times. When you consider that heart disease is the leading killer of Americans and is due, in part, to prolonged increased heart rate, blood pressure, and bad cholesterol, this becomes paramount to prolonged health. Consider, too, the second leading killer of Americans: cancer. One of the immune system's main jobs is to identify and eliminate cancerous tumors growing in the body. If you have stress hormones coursing throughout your body for too long, your immune system weakens, and that allows cancer to grow unchecked. Lastly, think of diabetes—the third leading cause of death in the U.S.—and the fact that stress hormones allow blood sugar levels to run rampant. Once again to quote Dr. Chestnut:

> "Without proper mechanoreception/nociception to your brain, you are literally sick and aging at an accelerated rate."

I hope you better understand how devastating it is to let your spine enter and progress through the Vicious Cycle. Not only does it rob your back and neck of their ability to be pain-free, but also, if left unchecked, can steal your potential to be healthy.

Chapter 21

How Long Does All This Take?

If time is not working for you, it's working against you.
—Anonymous

How long does it take to before you're caught deep within the Vicious Cycle? That's a good question. Considering the number of steps in the Vicious Cycle, you might think it takes a long time to get to the Point of No Return. Indeed, the answer may well surprise you.

The creation of a Buckling Point occurs in milliseconds (nearly instantaneous), and so does its recovery. I have found no absolute guidelines regarding the number of times one must use the spine poorly (or, for that matter, to what specific magnitude an impact must have) to force someone into the Dysfunctional Phase. I suspect this information is exceedingly hard to obtain because of the variables (age, nutrition, etc.) of recovery we've already discussed.

All else aside, once the Tipping Point has been crossed, you have precious little time.

- Scar tissue begins to be deposited immediately upon joint dysfunction,[3]
- After about a week, joint destruction begins,[4]
- In just two weeks, bone damage, cartilage deterioration, and bone spurring is detectable on X-ray,[3] and
- Within four weeks, irreversible bone spurring occurs.[4]

Here's the takeaway point: *after a Buckling Point has been created, you have less than four weeks to stop the Vicious Cycle.* So if you haven't had your back and neck professionally checked for dysfunction within the month, you're due.

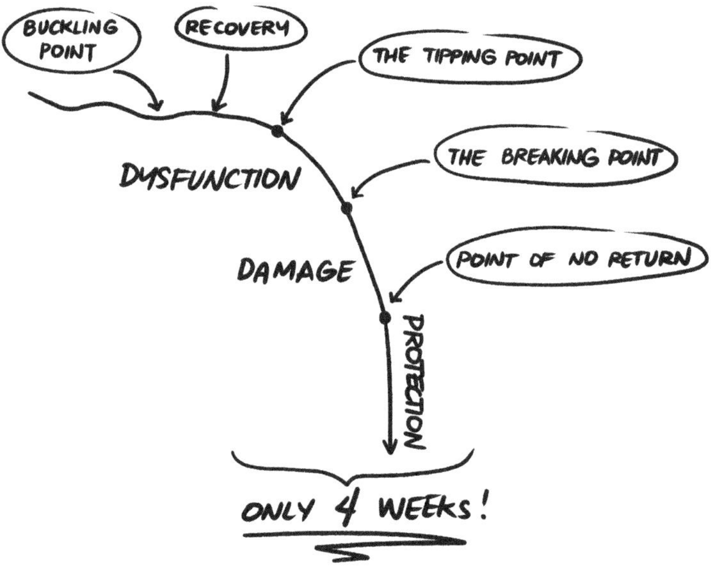

How Can This Happen So Quickly?

The Vicious Cycle starts slowly, and then accelerates faster and faster.

Here's an analogy. If your car is out-of-alignment, what happens to your tires? Do they wear down slower or faster? *Faster.* Now, when your tires wear down, what does that do to your car's alignment? Make it better or worse? *Worse.* Now that your car's alignment is worse, what does that mean for your tires? *They wear down much faster.* Which means what for the alignment? *It gets even worse.* You see, the tire's damage is progressively worsening. That final mile right before your tires blow out actually wears them down faster than all the miles that preceded it.

This is how the Vicious Cycle behaves—kind of like a snowball gathering in size and speed as it rolls down a hill. When dysfunction gets bad enough, it turns into destruction. As the tissues become damaged, what do you think happens to the degree of dysfunction? Does it get better or worse? *Worse.* What does it mean for the amount of damage that dysfunction is causing? Less or More? *More.* What does that do to the dysfunction? *Makes it worse.*

Not only do the nerves, muscles, and joints feed off of each other, but so do the phases of degradation. And although the first step into The Vicious Cycle is merely a stumble, a mistake, if your course isn't set right, the farther down you'll go and as the slope becomes steeper, the less time you have and the more likely you are to hurt and be in pain. This is why the old adage, "The worse the problem gets, the worse the problem gets" is true.

Chapter 22

Stopping the Vicious Cycle

There is a difference between knowledge and action.
—Dr. John Grams, pastor, and all around great dad

I've hit you with a lot of information, but it's all vital stuff to know. Think about it.

If *You Do Something Wrong* or if *Something Bad Happens To You* then comes:

- **The Buckling Point.** Nociception. Muscle imbalance. Abnormal joint movement.
- **The Tipping Point.** Constant nociception. Muscle incoordination. Turning off the pump.
- **The Breaking Point.** Sensitization. Stabilizer atrophy. Degeneration.
- **The Point of No Return.** Allodynia. Hyperalgesia. Neoneuralization. Scar tissue. Bone spurring.
- **The Dead Canary.** Pain. Nociceptive bombardment. Adaptive physiology. Sickness. Disease. Death.

Whew. That's a lot to grab hold of and swallow. But take heart: it's nothing like the physical pain I'm going to help you avoid.

When your body gets caught in The Vicious Cycle, you're able to do less and less. Your self-reliance and independence begins to crumble. You lose control of your body and life. Doing what you want becomes harder and harder. And for most people, The Vicious Cycle continues as they pile on Tylenol, NSAIDs, potions, lotions, injections, incomplete physical care, some type of cleverly marketed cure-all, and who knows, maybe a dreaded spinal surgery. Then, because The Vicious Cycle still hasn't been stopped, they go back to the doctor seeking answers, and hear the despicable soul-destroying words (and yes they're worth repeating), "There's nothing you can do about it," or "You'll have to learn to live with it," or "It's just a part of getting older," or "It's all in your head."

The thing that really grinds my gears, the thing that truly boggles my mind, is that during the whole cycle, the back and neck have always had the potential to get better. Your body is designed to fight back. Your body hates The Vicious Cycle. It hates that it's being forced to damage itself. It hates not being able to express its full potential. It hates not living a pain-free life. It desperately wants to recover.

All we have to do is to figure out how to give it what it wants.

Right now you know more about the actual origins of back and neck pain than most health professionals do. Good, but it's not good enough. Growing up my father always said, "Benjamin, there is a difference between knowledge and action," and he's right. It's how you apply this knowledge to your life that is the important part. Doing something different to get a different result is where the magic lies. But what do you do now? How do you break free of the Vicious Cycle and catapult yourself into a pain-free life?

Good question. Read on, my friend.

SECTION 5

Discover the Solution: A Commonsense and Scientifically Proven Method to Eliminate Back And Neck Pain[§]

Always look at the solution, not the problem. Learn to focus on what will give results.—Anonymous

[§]This section is not intended as a substitute for the medical advice of a physician. The reader should consult a physician in matters relating to his/her health before entering into treatment or making any changes to a current treatment plan.

Chapter 23

The Main Thing

The main thing is to keep the main thing, the main thing.
—Stephen Covey, author "The Seven Habits of Highly Effective People"

Becoming pain-free. That's the goal. We know what doesn't do it—drugs, surgery, and falling prey to pain myths. We know what the purpose of pain is, and how it develops in the back and neck. Now, it's time to leverage that knowledge and take the next step. In order to do so, however, you must understand one main thing.

Some things in this life are simply true. The sun rises in the east and sets in the west. You reap what you sow. One plus one equals two. See, it doesn't matter if you believe they're true or not, they simply are. They are as undeniable as they are unstoppable. Like if you don't *believe* in gravity, and then jump off a building, you're still going to fall.

With what I'm about to share with you, this is the case. There is a "truth" about back and neck pain, and if you take away only one thing from this entire book, it should be this: in order for your back and neck to be as pain-free as possible, they have to be as healthy as possible.

As Pain Free As Possible = As Healthy As Possible

But before we talk about what it means for the back and neck to be *"As Healthy as Possible,"* we must first know what health is. In a dictionary you will find that health is defined as, "The state of an organism when it functions optimally without evidence of disease." The key words are "optimally" and "functions." When something functions optimally, it means it's working at 100 percent. For the spine, it's the state in which the nerves, muscles, and joints are working as good as they possibly can be. The Vicious Cycle robs you of that and relentlessly pulls your spine away from peak performance—away from being healthy—and closer to pain.

Then: *As Healthy As Possible = Optimal Function*

Now, one system in the body is responsible for making sure every other system in the body is functioning optimally: The Nervous System. It supervises and coordinates the activity of every cell, tissue, and organ at breakneck speed and with astounding precision. Its complexity is mind boggling, and its architecture is awe-inspiring. One of my wise professors would say, "The human nervous system is the apex of creation in the known universe" and I agree. If you think about it, you probably agree as well.

Despite its grandeur, the setup of the nervous system is very simple. The brain sends messages down the spinal cord and out through the nerves, telling whatever is on the end of that nerve—heart, lungs, stomach, or muscle—how to function optimally. How well the body is able to function is really dependent on the messages the brain sends. This means that in order for the body to function optimally, the output of the brain also has to be optimal.

Optimal Function = Optimal Brain Output

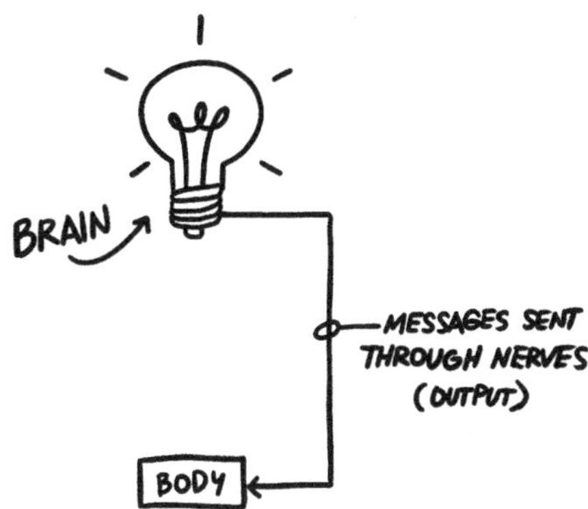

But how does the brain know what to do? For instance, if you're walking up a flight of stairs, how does the brain know to send messages to the heart to beat faster and to the lungs to breathe deeper? How does the brain know to regulate your blood sugar? How does it know to get your skin to sweat when you're hot? The answer is that the body tells the brain what's happening to it, once again, through the nerves, and then the brain interprets that information and responds accordingly.

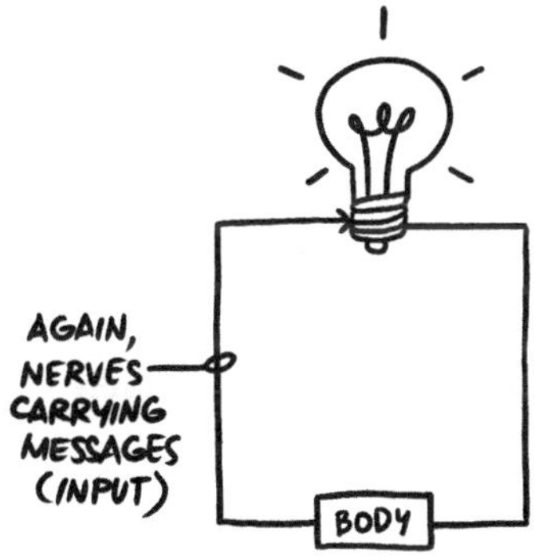

Then, in order for the brain to control the body really well (optimal output), it must receive really good and complete information from the body. So,

Optimal Output = Optimal Input

I know I'm getting a little technical, but stick with me here. Like I said, this is *the* most important concept of this book.

In some systems in the body, this input/output happens automatically; meaning, we have no conscious control over it. Take the immune system. You cannot consciously tell your immune system to start fighting bacteria or viruses. It just does it. Nerves detect the invaders, alert the brain, and then the brain triggers an immune response. The digestive system is another example. You cannot, right now, by the force of willpower, make your stomach produce more acid—no way. Only once food enters the stomach, and the nerves detect it, does acid start getting released to break down the food. It's the same with the cardiovascular system as well as the skin system. If you get a paper cut, no matter how hard you think and stare at your bleeding finger, it's not going to heal any faster. All of the systems of the body run on autopilot, but the neuromusculoskeletal system is an exception.

It almost goes without saying that you have at least some control over your body. You can lift your arm, close your eyelids, hold your breath, and bend to pick up things. But just because we initiate the action by willing it, doesn't mean we really control it. Here's what I mean.

> *The mechanisms that go into planning and executing a movement are far more complex than the brain simply issuing a command and the nerves executing it.*
>
> *For example, suppose that you go to pick up a glass of water*

that you think is cool and refreshing, but is actually boiling hot. As soon as you touch the glass, you immediately pull your hand back, by reflex, without thinking about it.

But suppose that next your child tries to grab this glass, which you already know is hot. In this case, because your child's safety is so important to you, you can consciously overcome the reflex to pull your hand away. Instead, using your voluntary muscle control, you grab the glass yourself and put it where your child can't reach it.

Lastly, if someone tells you that the glass is made of fine crystal and not ordinary glass, you will probably handle it more carefully. In other words, your brain will take this information into account and adapt your method of grasping the glass accordingly.

All of these facts demonstrate that the execution of a movement is not simply a matter of the brain's sending a "Go!" command through the nerves but is rather the result of a highly elaborate construct. Moreover, the remarkable adaptability of movement demonstrates the involvement of powerful mechanisms.[1]

Yes, we do have some say in how we move, but the majority of motions themselves—the speed, force, timing, coordination, etc.—are on autopilot. The part of the brain that controls this is called the cerebellum. It's located at the base of your skull, and is impressively chock-full of nerves that's sole purpose is to make sure you're moving optimally.

Following what we've already discussed, in order for your brain to ensure that your back and neck are functioning optimally, it needs as much information about your spine as possible. Like how the joints are positioned, how they're moving, how fast they're moving, and how much stress is on them because of that movement.

Now, in the last section we covered the type of nerves that do this. Do you remember? Mechanoreceptors. Your brain needs as much mechanoreception as possible in order to ensure your back and neck are functioning optimally.

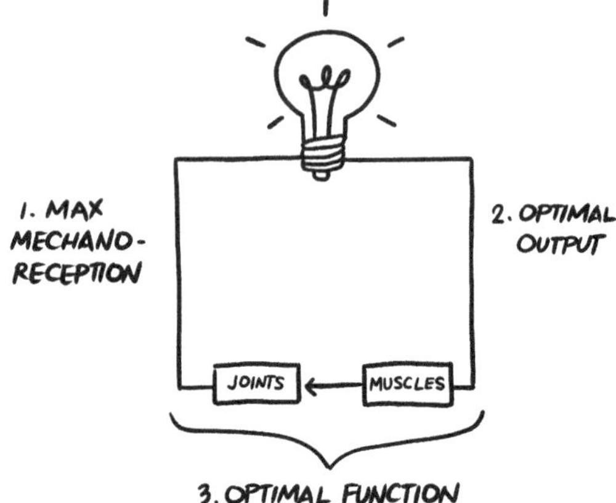

But what about the nociceptors? You know, the "bad guys" of the entire Vicious Cycle? For the intents and purposes of this chapter, nociception should really be considered as "no-mechanoreception." Meaning that if nociceptors are firing, the mechanoreceptors are not. Then, if the mechanoreceptors aren't firing, the brain becomes disconnected from knowing what the joints are doing. Nociception is bad input.

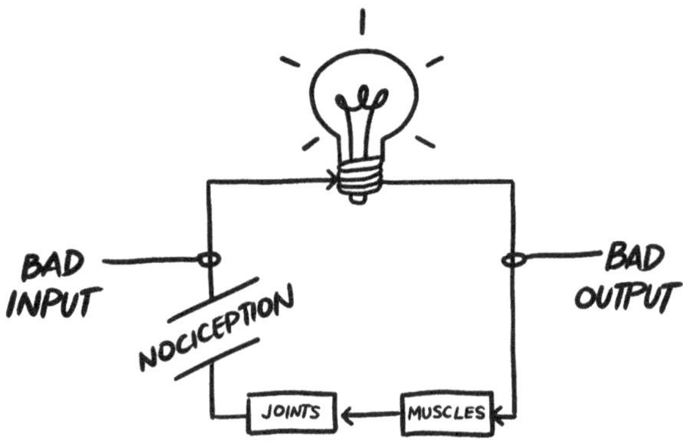

For the back and neck, optimal input is when mechanoreception is maximized and nociception is minimized.**

Optimal Input = Maximal Mechanoreception and Minimal Nociception

The next question then is: how do you do this? How do you ensure that your brain is getting optimal input for optimal output? This is where it gets exciting. Muscles, tendons, and ligaments—the things that hold joints together—are full of mechanoreceptors. They're not only responsible for controlling a joint's movement, but also for containing it within its normal limits. Joints must move as fully as possible, and at the same time, not exceed their normal limits (i.e., no Buckling Points)—that's how you get optimal input to the brain (your cerebellum to be precise).

Maximal Mechanoreception and Minimal Nociception =Joints Moving As Good As Possible

But it doesn't end there. In order for joints to move as good as possible, they must have two things: 1) Optimal alignment and 2) Balance between the two muscle groups.

Joints Moving As Good As Possible = Optimal Alignment + Muscle Balance

That's the bottom line. If you can keep your spine in good alignment when you sit, lift, bend, sleep, stand, or whatever, and keep the deep Stabilizers balanced with the superficial Movers, your spine will be as healthy as possible, making it as pain-free as possible.

**For the other spinal geeks out there reading this, I do not mean absolutely no nociception. Some, I imagine, is good for us, like red wine. But also like red wine, too much will cause problems.

This line of logic stripped to its barest elements looks like this:

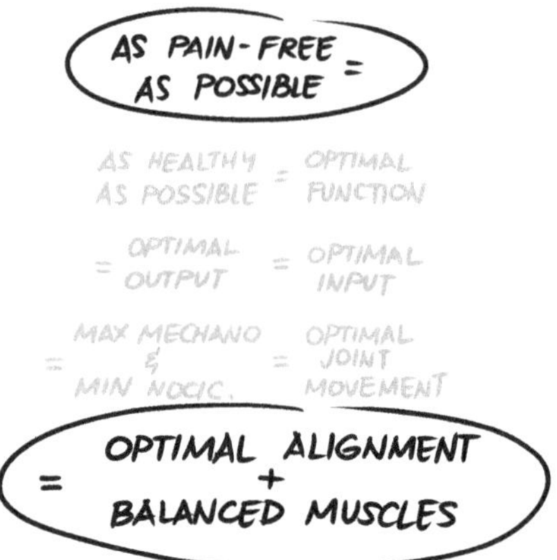

This is what The Solution does. It doesn't simply operate within this framework—it maximizes it. Which is why, as you're about to find out, it is the most effective way to rid the back and neck of pain. By the way, guess what doesn't operate within this framework, or at best, leverages it incompletely? Standard medical care, pain management clinics, and the vast majority of physical medicine. As a healthcare field, *we have failed to keep the main thing the main thing.* Many other things—technological advances, money, and political power, to name a few—have replaced the main thing: *getting and keeping people healthy.* This is why people are suffering from so much pain. It's time for a better approach to pain. It's time for a better answer: The Solution.

Summary

#4 OPTIMAL INPUT
(MAX MECHANO. MIN. NOCI.)
#3 OPTIMAL MOVEMENT
#5 OPTIMAL OUTPUT
JOINTS
MUSCLES
#2 OPTIMAL ALIGNMENT
#1 IN BALANCE
#6 OPTIMAL FUNCTION
#7 AS HEALTHY AS POSSIBLE
#8 AS PAIN-FREE AS POSSIBLE

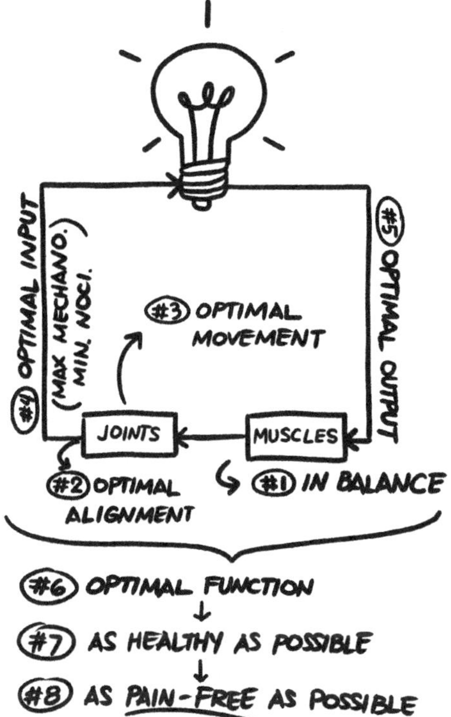

Chapter 24

THE SOLUTION
Part 1: Spinal Adjustments

As knowledge is acquired, it must be organized and put into use, for a definite purpose, through practical plans. Knowledge has no value except that which can be gained from its application toward some worthy end.—Napoleon Hill

There's great potential in the bond between joints, nerves, and muscles. For example, if the Tipping Point is crossed, this connection powers the Vicious Cycle, bringing your back and neck to ruin, and you as close to pain-full as possible.

But what if I told you there is a way to flip the script? A way to redirect this power? A way to reverse the Vicious Cycle? A way to shift from the breaking down of your spine—Tipping Points, Breaking Points, and Points of No Return—to the building up of your spine—*a Turning Point?* That would be great news, and would salvage and heal your back and neck, and would get you pain-free. That, ladies and gentlemen, is The Solution.

Beginning the Turnaround: The Joints

The mast of a sailboat is the tall piece of lumber right in the center of the ship. It provides the means for the wind and sail to propel the vessel through the water. A mast can be buffeted by a storm, but as long as it does not break, the sailboat will be able to carry on. If the mast does break, it's big trouble because the very thing that gave the sailboat the ability to sail would be lost.

Your spine is much like a mast. It's right in the center of your body and it provides the means for your central nervous system and muscles to propel you through life. Buckling Points can occur without consequence as long as they recover. However, if a Buckling Point does not recover it's big trouble because the very thing that keeps your spine healthy and pain-free—optimal joint movement—would be lost, thrusting your back and neck into the Vicious Cycle.

The good news is that *the way into the Vicious Cycle is also the way out.*

Once the joints become dysfunctional, they begin losing mobility. As this worsens, the nutrient pump they control starts shutting down, starving bone and cartilage of vital nutrients. Now the joints begin to self-destruct—cartilage cells begin to die, and bone deteriorates. Invariably, this leads to things like degeneration, stenosis, bone spurs, and more forms of arthritis than you can imagine—and all because the joints don't move correctly.

This is where The Solution intervenes. It turns *dysfunction* and *damage* into *function* and *healing* by doing one thing: restoring mobility. That's right. The first step in becoming pain-free is to get the joints moving optimally again. Why is this the first step? Because by restoring motion:

- **You turn on mechanoreceptors and turn off nociceptors.** This stops the sensitization process that leads to chronic pain. Not only that, but the nerve reflex leading to the muscle imbalance turns off, and this opens the doorway for the muscles to start to heal. Remember, the muscles can only get as good as the joints are, not the other way around. Last but not least, mechanoreceptors start sending normal messages to the brain, which removes a tremendous roadblock to your future health and vitality.
- **Your spinal cartilage begins to heal.** Motion gets the nutrient pump working again. And like water to a withering plant, the restored flow of nutrients into the cartilage sparks a healing process so effective that not only does it slow degenerative disc disease, bone spurring, and arthritis1, but it also heals herniated or torn discs.[2]
- **Your bone begins to rebuild.** Once again, because the nutrient pump is turned back on, the bone cells stop dying and start doing their jobs—building new bone!
- **You break up scar tissue.** The adhesions that have fused muscles, tendons, and joints together causing stiffness and nasty tightness, get busted up, like greasing a door's dry hinges.
- **You stimulate new muscle growth.** By the joints simply moving more, the muscles become more active, causing them to get stronger.
- **You lessen pain.** There's a reason why rubbing your head when you hit it makes you feel better. It's called the Pain-Gate Theory. It states that your brain can only handle so many messages at once, and if you flood the brain with a

message other than pain, you feel less pain. By rubbing your head, you are interfering with pain signals through the sensation of your skin. So, by restoring normal movement to your joints, you interfere with pain signals through mechanoreception. Cool, huh?

By the way, restoring optimal movement to the joints to stop the Vicious Cycle isn't something I came up with. It was written about long before my time. Here's what Dr. Charles Lantz, the director of research for Life Chiropractic College West, said back in 1990:

> *A vicious cycle has been described in which muscle tightness leads to joint dysfunction, which in turn leads to more muscle tightness and joint dysfunction; the specified treatment for this condition being to return joints to their full range-of-motion and maintain that range through the healing phases.* [3] (author paraphrase)

All in all, any of the damages that occur while joints are dysfunctional are reversible upon restoring optimal movement if you act fast enough. If you don't, and the back and neck enter into the Pathological Protection phase, you won't be able to undo all of the damage, but you can undo a lot.

You're never too late to get better than you are right now, but you have to take action.

What's the best way to do this?

You *could* inject the joints full of cortisone. You *could* take Tylenol, ibuprofen, Excedrin, or Aleve. Better yet, you *could* start popping prescription painkillers or muscle relaxants. Or you *could* hire a doctor with special technology to kill off nerves. *Maybe* you have surgery to either cut out the joint or fuse it all up—that way you don't have a dysfunctional joint anymore, right?

Wrong. Because they don't make the joint move better, doing any of those things is like a person feverishly mopping the floor while the faucet is still gushing water (if this analogy doesn't ring a bell, go back and re-read the end of Chapter 7). The most effective way to restore spinal range-of-motion is through spinal adjustments.[5,6,7]

How effective is spinal adjusting? Remember back to the first pain myth when I mentioned the "one part" of The Solution that was 500 times more effective than Vioxx and Celebrex? This is it! Furthermore, in the words of scientist and international authority on the spine, Dr. James Chestnut,

> *The **fact** is that the most evidence-based interventions for spine related disorders in terms of effectiveness, cost effectiveness, and safety are **chiropractic adjustments**, spinal fitness exercises, and lifestyle.* [8] (Emphasis mine.)

Why? Because adjustments directly address the Tipping Point of the Vicious Cycle: joint dysfunction. That's a really big deal.

Research Highlights

Now, before we dive any deeper, know that the evidence for adjustments is so extensive that we are only going to be able to hit the highlights here.

Pran Magna graduated from the University of Toronto with a PhD in economics. He has been a professor at the Telfer School of Management, teaching ethics, health economics, and globalization. He is also the director of the master's program in health administration. Pran is a really smart man. So much so that in 1993 the Canadian government's Ontario Ministry of Health commissioned him to evaluate chiropractic spinal adjustments for the management of low back pain (you'll learn why the word "chiropractic" is always linked with "adjustments" in a moment). What he wrote is called the Magna Report and, to date, it represents one of the largest existing analyses of scientific literature on low back pain.

In the report, he found:

> *Spinal adjustments applied by chiropractors are shown to be more effective than alternative treatments for low back pain. Many medical therapies are of questionable validity or are clearly inadequate.*

And that there is a "lack of any convincing argument or evidence to the contrary."

The Magna Report concluded:

In our view, there is a constellation of the evidence of

- *(a) the effectiveness and cost effectiveness of chiropractic management of low back pain.*
- *(b) the untested, questionable or harmful nature of many current medical therapies.*
- *(c) the economic efficiency of chiropractic care for low back pain compared to medical care.*
- *(d) the safety of chiropractic care.*
- *(e) the higher satisfaction levels expressed by patients under chiropractors.*

On top of that, more studies have proven that restoring full range of motion through specific spinal adjusting is not simply better and safer than standard medical care, but it is better than physical therapy, exercising, "back school," and acupuncture, too. It also blows surgery out of the water in both short and long-term outcomes.[9-13] Furthermore, it was found that people who had utilized spinal adjustments for pain "had fewer surgeries, used fewer opioids, and had lower costs for medical care," and the use of specific spinal adjustments, "achieves the best recovery rates, the lowest use of drugs, the least time off work, and is more cost-effective compared to drugs and physiotherapy directive active exercises."[14]

Hmmm. Enough said.

Where can you get this done?

You *could* get it done by a doctor of osteopathy, a doctor of chiropractic, or maybe a physical therapist. But, there's a reason why Dr. Pran said in his report that spinal adjustments when applied by a chiropractor are most effective, because he also found that "there is also some evidence to suggest that spinal manipulations are less safe and less effective when performed by non-chiropractic professionals."

Let's dig deeper.

First, doctors of osteopathy are good, smart people. I love osteopaths. If you're an osteopath and you're reading this, I love you, but you are not the best at spinal adjusting. A study published in the journal called Academic Medicine, in 2001, showed that less than 5 percent of osteopaths are actually still doing it in their practices.[15] That's not a lot.

Second, physical therapists are good, smart people. I love physical therapists. If you're a physical therapist and you're reading this, I love you, but you are not the best at spinal adjusting. Researchers have compared adjustments done by a physical therapist to those of a chiropractor, and found that being treated by a chiropractor was superior than that of a physical therapist.[10,16]

One research team went so far to say that "the advantage for chiropractic over conventional hospital treatment was not a trivial amount" and that "surprisingly, the difference was seen most strongly in patients with chronic symptoms." This means that the patients with the oldest and probably most stubborn pain got the most relief from being adjusted by a chiropractor, and not by a physical therapist.

Figuring out where you *could* get it done is a lot different than figuring out where you *should* get it done. You should get it done by a chiropractor. Here's why:

It is uncontestable that chiropractors have, by far, spent the most time being trained on adjusting techniques, and also have the most advanced methods of evaluation. Out of all the professions discussed, chiropractors simply spend the most time doing this therapy. For example, a very conservative estimate is that I have performed 500 spinal adjustments per week, every week, for the past five years of practice, which comes to over 100,000 adjustments in my career. That's a lot of time in the trenches. Knowing what I know about the back and neck, seeing people suffer with back and neck pain the way that I have, having to deal with my own problems with back and neck pain, and receiving regular spinal care for about seven years, I wouldn't trust anyone other than a well-trained, smart, and clinically competent chiropractor to adjust my spine. Ever.

For Best Results, Use as Directed

- **Don't beat around the bush.** Let's be clear on what won't fix joint dysfunction and lack of range of motion: spinal surgery, pain medications, and injections. And naturally based things like icing, heating, essential oils, taping, and compression sleeves won't do it either. These practices all help reduce inflammation, but they do not directly address joint dysfunction.

- **Stay on target.** A human spine has twenty-four joints where a Buckling Point could occur and each one of those joints has the potential to be dysfunctional in any combination of twelve different directions. Adding another layer of complexity to this, each one of those joints also has a unique set of characteristics that dictate exactly how it should be adjusted. For example, the top vertebrae in your neck need to be adjusted differently than the lowest vertebrae in your back. The person you go to needs to have the ability to figure all this out. Based on their extensive training, chiropractors have the most advanced methods to do just that.
- **Not all range-of-motion treatment is created equally.** Not every type of treatment can restore range of motion and decrease pain as effectively as adjustments. Stretching won't do it. Yoga, Pilates, and CrossFit won't do it. Mobilization techniques like the use of a foam roller won't do it. Physical therapy and massages won't do it.[17,18,19,20,21] Don't get me wrong—all of these things are good for your back and neck, and they certainly can help improve range of motion, but they cannot *fully* restore it. And remember, that's the key: to *fully* restore the joints' range of motion. Only spinal adjustments can get that done.

Conclusion

Restoring mobility through specific spinal adjustments is like repairing a broken mast and hoisting it on your sailboat. It's a good start, but the job doesn't end there. Once it's up, it needs to be anchored and stabilized. And that's exactly what needs to happen to your spine next if you're ever to get pain-free.

Chapter 25

The Solution
Part 2: Spinal Exercise

I really regret that workout.—No One Ever

When you use your back and neck incorrectly, or *Something Bad Happens To You,* a Buckling Point is created, and muscles that were once your spine's biggest protector become its greatest threat. That has to change to get out of pain. You must get your muscles on your side once again.

Here's how.

The Deep, Spinal Stabilizers

Once the Tipping Point has been crossed, life becomes difficult for the deep Stabilizers. At first, because of inhibition, their reaction time is slowed and their coordination begins to wane. Eventually, some of them stop being used completely. This lack of use turns into weakness. Weakness brings destruction. After a while, the muscles and the parts of the brain that control them begin to die off, which is not a pretty picture.

What do you do about it? Turn lack-of-use into lots-of-use by forcing the deep Stabilizers to become active. This turns weakness into strength, destruction into reconstruction, and your dead muscles will be raised to life. The use of these muscles will force your brain to grow new neurons, reestablishing its control. Coordination will be restored. Reaction time will improve. You'll feel stronger, move better, have more balance, and most importantly, have less pain.

What's the best way to get this done? Through spinal exercises. And like with spinal adjusting, the research and data on exercise relieving back and neck pain is so extensive that it's almost mind numbing. Here, again, are highlights.

Research Highlights

In 1992, some 103 low-back pain sufferers were randomly assigned into a carefully graded exercise program. Others in the group were given "the usual" care (ice and rest). All were blue-collar workers on sick leave for disability because of their low back pain. This study found that the people who received exercise training returned to work faster than those who did not.[22] Duh! Of course people who were given the means to directly address one of the components of the Vicious Cycle got better. Study[23], after study[24], after study[25], after study[26], after study[27] proves this. Another study was done in 2010 that involved over 6,000 people that showed the same thing.[28] Yep, the science is abundantly clear that if you're suffering from back and neck pain, you need to be exercising your deep Stabilizers.

Interestingly, spinal exercises not only relieve pain but also stop and reverse weakness, destruction, and the muscle death that happens to them in the Vicious Cycle. Case in point: An Australian study that showed if low back pain patients perform exercises, the atrophy of a deep Stabilizer (called the Multifidus) was prevented.[29]

Why does exercising the spinal Stabilizers work so consistently well? It's simple. When you keep the deep Stabilizers strong they do their job at holding the joints together and protecting them. You don't have to be a genius to understand that. So if you're suffering from back and/or neck pain and not doing spinal exercises, you're missing a big part of what it takes to be pain-free.

Where can you find how to exercise your deep, spine-stabilizing muscles?

Once again, for some reason beyond me, more doctors haven't figured this out so you may have to do some work in order to find a good back-and-neck rehab program. This is not an all-inclusive list by any means, but doctors of chiropractic, physical therapists, and occupational therapists are going to be your best bet. The key is to know what you're seeking. If the typical program of the person you're seeing is a handful of "one-size-fits-all" sessions, and then you're sent home with a grainy printout of exercises straight out of the 1980s, run for the hills.

For Best Results, Use as Directed:

- **Be picky!** Not all exercises are created equal. If you wanted to improve your heart health, you would do cardiovascular exercise like jogging. If you wanted to build whole-body strength, you would focus on weight lifting. If you wanted to work on your stability, you would do balance-reinforcing exercises. You see, different types of exercise give different results. When it comes to relieving your back and neck pain, the exercises you perform need to strengthen the deep spinal Stabilizers which can only be done through certain exercises. Walking, jogging, staying active, and lifting weights are all good things to do for your health, but they aren't the right kind of exercise to get your back and neck out of the Vicious Cycle.

- **Specificity is key.** The exercises need to be done in a very specific manner. The truth is your back and neck can be exercised in a variety of ways, but, based on your pain level, body type, and progression through the Vicious Cycle, only the right way *for you* will get your pain gone. The "one-exercise-fits-all" approach to getting the spine pain-free is hogwash. In fact, one study showed that the more specific the exercises are, the better the results.[30] You might think this is common sense, but you'd be surprised how many physical medicine professionals seem to have forgotten about this.
- **Coaching is a must.** The farther down your spine the Vicious Cycle has gotten, the harder it's going to be to actually turn on the deep Stabilizers because the nerves controlling them get damaged, making the brain/muscle connection weak. On top of that, the superficial Movers are hyperactively trying to take over the Stabilizer's job. This makes it impossible to be able to exercise your Stabilizers in the right way all by yourself. As it is with so many things in life, practice does *not* make perfect—only *perfect* practice makes perfect. Having an outside set of expert eyes train you, critique you, and give you feedback as you perform the exercises makes it possible for you to strengthen your Stabilizers to their fullest potential.

- **Strength first, endurance second.** Stabilizers are used all the time. Even when you're asleep, they're being used. You can't get complacent by only getting them strong, you have to build up their endurance. They have to get strong and stay strong over a long period of time to keep you out of pain.
- **Muscle memory takes time.** Learning how to do these exercises comes in three stages. If you've ever played an instrument, this will make perfect sense. *The first stage is where you understand what you have to do, but you simply can't do it.* In learning to play piano, for instance, understanding where your fingers need to land is entirely different from being able to get them to do so. At this point, you lack muscle coordination and strength. The only way to change that is through practice, patience, and time. There is no way to get around it. That's the first stage of learning back-and-neck exercises—you understand what you should be doing, and you start working on being able to do it.

  At some point, you'll be able to strike the key at the right time and with the right finger, but it still takes a lot of con centration and effort. *The second stage is you're able to do it, but you really have to think about it.*

  Once you're here, you have to continue to push your muscles. More practice. More repetition. More time. More coaching. Keep repeating this until you meet *the third and final stage—where you do it without thinking.* You'll be like the master pianist whose fingers effortlessly grace the keys. The beautiful thing about getting to this point is that once you're there, you really won't have to think too much about your back and neck. Remember, the deep Stabilizers are involuntary muscles. In the Vicious Cycle, this works against you because once they start shutting down, they're hard to stop. In the healing process, this works for you because all you have to do is feed them an occasional exercise session, and they take care of the rest. It's a beautiful, very pain-free place to be.

- **Don't stop until you get enough.** These exercises will take you a long way toward achieving flexibility, strength, and coordination, but it can't stop there. These need to become a habit, and you have to continue long after the pain has lessened or perhaps disappeared completely. Stopping these exercises is like sending pain an invitation back into your life.
- **Less is best.** While you're on your way to getting pain-free, you might be told that you'll need big, expensive, technologically advanced machines to strengthen the Stabilizers. Wrong. The best spinal rehab is done low-tech, and these things will do the trick: a yoga mat, gym ball, a couple of weights, and wall bands.
- **Consistency is vital.** Who has the healthier set of teeth? The person who brushes once a week or the person who brushes daily? Duh. So it is with your Stabilizers. Doing the exercises once a day, every day, is better for you than doing a session once a week because it constantly reminds the Stabilizers how they should be behaving. Once a day, every day—that's your quota.

Conclusion

Through spinal adjustments, the joints have started moving fully, and through spinal exercise, the Stabilizers have gotten stronger. At this point, it's like the broken mast has been repaired and secured. What needs to be done now is to hoist the anchor and set sail. To accomplish this, another component of the Vicious Cycle must be taken care of—the superficial Movers.

Chapter 26

The Solution
Part 3: Hands-on Muscle Therapy

Nothing is so healing as the human touch.—Bobby Fischer, very first American born chess world champion

During the Vicious Cycle, the Movers play a sinister role. Here's what I mean. Joint dysfunction and Stabilizer weakness are what push the back and neck through the Vicious Cycle. But the Movers do something different. They do not *push.* Instead, they *hold.* Like the teeth of a ratchet, the Movers stop the spine from being able to go any other way except deeper into the Vicious Cycle.

The Superficial Movers

After the Tipping Point, because of facilitation, the Movers become hyperactive.Then, whereas the Stabilizers start wasting away because of lack of use, and the Movers start tightening because of overuse. They become short and contracted and begin micro-tearing and scarring, causing the notorious muscle knots everyone seems to complain about. Ultimately, by the final phase of the Vicious Cycle, they are so weak and short that they become a source of pain all on their own.

How do you break Movers out of the Vicious Cycle?

Like this.

Imagine you've been given a beautiful piece of land to live on for the rest of your life. But there's a catch: you cannot live anywhere else except on that land. It's a great spot, but it's the only one you're getting. On this land is an old, ugly house. The foundation is cracked, the support beams are splitting, and the shingles are rotten. It's in complete disrepair. While you do have to keep the land, there are no rules about having to keep the house. What would you do? That's right, grab a sledgehammer, rent a bulldozer, and demolish it. Why? Because *sometimes you have to tear down before you can build up.*

And so it is with the Movers—they're the only ones you've been given, but there's no reason why you can't remodel them. The scar tissue must be broken down, the adhesions busted up, and the contracted tissue, lengthened. By doing this, you will give them (and yourself) an opportunity to rebuild, heal, and become pain-free.

The best way to do this is through hands-on muscle therapy. Like with the other interventions, the research on the effectiveness of hands-on muscle therapy (generally referred to as massage) and pain relief isn't up for debate. Here are the highlights.

Research Highlights:

- Massage relieves chronic pain, chronic pain of moderate-to-severe intensity, and helps those with myalgia.[31,32,33]
- Massage improves subjective perception of and function for those with Carpal Tunnel Syndrome.[34]

- Muscle-specific massage therapy is effective for reducing the incidence of chronic tension headaches.[35]
- In one interesting study done in 2007, researchers looked at eight trials of massage therapy and found that it was as effective as exercise, and a little more effective than acupuncture.[36]

Basically, all of these articles say that breaking down muscle knots and scar tissue adhesions in the superficial Movers will help you feel less pain. This theme is so common in the literature that here's a quote pulled directly from an instructional course to orthopedic surgeons: "Massage decreases symptoms and improves function."[37] And that's the key—you have to get the Movers to function better, making them healthier; then you'll be as close to pain-free as possible.

For Best Results, Use as Directed

"The right type of muscle therapy applied to the right spot, on the right muscle, at the right time." —Ben Grams, DC

"The right type"—If you're trying to demolish a wall, you need a sledgehammer, not a rake. And so it is with muscle therapy. Some techniques, like "Light Touch" massage, are designed to release endorphins—natural pain killers that the body houses—and not bust up scar tissue adhesions. That's not what we're seeking. When it comes to getting the Movers out of the Vicious Cycle, an aggressive massage is needed. Now, breaking down scar tissue should be a bit sore and uncomfortable, so if you're on the table and the massage you're getting "hurts so good," you're probably on the right track. A few techniques that fit within this category are:

deep tissue, cross friction, Active Release Technique, Graston, and myofascial release.

"The right spot"—Specificity is key. Not only does the right muscle need to be worked, but the right spot on the right muscle needs to be worked on. Here's a couple tips:

A very important spot in a muscle is something called the musculotendinous junction, which is right where the muscle turns into a tendon before it attaches onto a bone. This is the weakest part of the muscle because it is an area of transition. The tissues there aren't fully muscle, and they aren't fully tendon. They're more half-and-half, which means they have half the strength. Unfortunately, it's also where a large amount of stress ends up when you use the muscles. The combination of these two things makes it fertile ground for the growth of scar tissue.

The other spot, that is commonly overlooked, but where scar tissue loves to grow is between muscles. You see, the Movers are layered and typically glide over each other without problem. But when scar tissue forms between the layers, it adheres them to each other, and keeps your muscles all knotted up. If you could see it, it would look like two old books on a shelf with a thick spider web between them.

Most hands-on muscle therapy, especially when done by nonprofessionals, or when employing most do-it-yourself muscle widgets, you cannot directly treat these areas because they're difficult to reach and hard to find. The muscle/tendon junction, for example, can be located underneath the bone they attach onto. To get as close to pain-free as possible, with extreme precision, hands-on muscle therapy needs to be applied to the right spot. In fact, entire textbooks are written about the necessity of being on the right spot, how to find it, and what to do once you're there. One book I refer to quite often has over 750 pages, and has more detail than you can shake a stick at.

"The right muscle"—Sometimes muscle pain isn't as straightforward as it seems. In the world of physical medicine, it's well known that the muscle *feeling* the pain isn't always the one that is *causing* the pain. This phenomenon is called "referred pain." The mechanics of how this happens isn't really important here. What is important is that it happens, it's common, and in order to get pain-free, you can't afford to be thrown off by this.

"The right time"—When one Mover gets damaged and forms scar tissue, a second Mover has to compensate. Soon that muscle gets overworked, damaged, and forms scar tissue. Causing a third Mover to do the same. This destruction spreads while the first Mover, where it all began, progressively worsens. This is why finding and treating the right muscle is so important.

The Mover that's been beat up the most is the one that has to be cleared out first. Why? Because that muscle is like a slow driver in the fast lane—it's causing a long line of issues to build up behind it. Until that muscle gets fixed, none of the other muscles can get as good as they should. Once you do clear that one up though, it's truly a beautiful thing. Each subsequent muscle clears up with increasing ease. And before you know it, the slow driver has switched lanes, opening up the road ahead of you. You press the accelerator and move yourself that much closer to being pain-free.

All-in-all, *any* type of hands-on muscle therapy applied *anywhere* on *probably* the right muscle at *any* time could be good in the short run, but will be bad in the long run. It may help you relax and provide some relief, but if your goal is to break the bonds of the Vicious Cycle, hands-on muscle therapy must be applied to the right spot, on the right muscle, at the right time.

Lastly…

- **Stretch with the massage.** The breaking down of scar tissue activates the body's healing mechanisms, and immediately new muscle starts getting laid down. This is a prime opportunity to tell the body that the Movers need to be remade in a longer and stronger way. Remember, Movers get their strength from being able to contract, and when they get knotted up, they lose that ability, becoming weak. The best way to stimulate those muscles on how you want them to grow is by being stretched. This window of opportunity doesn't last very long so it needs to be done in a timely manner, preferably immediately following a scar tissue-breakdown session.
- **Get someone else's help.** We need to make an important point here. In our day and age, there are tons of "at home," do-it-yourself, muscle gizmos that you *could* purchase, but that doesn't mean you *should*. Let me be perfectly clear: all of these things have their place, but they are not specific enough to get you out of the Vicious Cycle—and out of pain. You're going to need the help of a trained professional to do that. Once you're out of pain, those things are a great way to help yourself stay well.

So where can you go to get this?

Looking at a provider's professional credentials is a good place to start, but doesn't guarantee they understand the details of The Solution. Professional credentials are the letters after someone's name.

For example, mine are "Ben Grams, D.C." which stands for Doctor of Chiropractic.

But just because someone is trained as a chiropractor doesn't automatically mean he or she knows how to deliver this type of hands-on muscle therapy. Same holds true about P.T. (Physical Therapists), M.D. (Doctors of Medicine), D.O. (Doctors of Osteopathy), L.A.c. (Licensed Acupuncturists), L.M.T (Licensed Massage Therapists), or O.T.s (Occupational Therapists). Plus, healthcare professionals can get certifications that add even more letters to their name making it difficult to figure out who you should go to. Instead of diving into each one, let's keep it simple.

When you first meet this professional, ask how scar tissue forms in muscles (through overuse and micro-tearing). Then ask what specifically he is going to do about it (like use a special tool, stretching, or hands-on technique to break it down). If he can answer those two questions with confidence, then you're probably on the right track.

By getting hands-on muscle therapy and following these guidelines, the anchor keeping you in the Vicious Cycle will be hoisted and your ship will be ready to set sail to the land of no pain.

Once you begin that journey, how do you ensure that you arrive at a pain-free destination and never return to the deep, dangerous waters of the Vicious Cycle? The answer to this is found in the pages to follow.

Chapter 27

THE SOLUTION
Part 4: Training

Give a man to fish and you feed him for a day. Teach a man to fish and you feed him for a lifetime.—Chinese proverb

Let's review what you've learned so far. Spinal adjusting, spinal exercises, and hands-on muscle therapy are very effective treatments for back and neck pain. Not only that, they're incredibly less expensive and safer than medications and surgery.

Pretty impressive, but it's not good enough. Why? Because good is enough is *never* good enough. I want to deliver to you the *most* effective treatment for back and neck pain—The Solution—but before I can do that I need to unveil one more component.

You might be thinking: "What's wrong with what you've laid out? That treatment sounds like the winning ticket." The answer is just that—spinal adjustments, spinal exercises, and hands-on muscle therapy are *treatment.* They only address the dysfunction once it's set in. They only repair what has already been damaged. They only slow the pathological protective changes once they've occurred. But what if you get all the way to your desired destination—to the point of being without pain—and then you unwittingly create another Buckling Point in your spine and cross the Tipping Point? That's right; you'll be pulled back in the Vicious Cycle faster than you can say ouch."

The problem with what we've discussed in this section so far is that it's all treatment. Spinal adjustments, spinal exercise, and hands-on muscle therapy only treat problems that are already there. They do not *prevent* problems from occurring. Said differently, up to this point, I've shown you what the most effective mops are, where to find them, and how to best use them to clean up the mess, but I have not yet shown you how to turn off the faucet—which, in my opinion, is the *most* important component of The Solution.

Mistakes and Buckling Points

Imagine a really bad driver. He comes to a screeching halt at every stop sign and then accelerates like a bat out of hell. He never slows down to take corners, and redlines the engine every chance he gets. And to top it off, he's never changed the oil, replaced fluids, or had the "check engine" light looked at. One day, while driving like a maniac, his car violently lurches forward, then abruptly stops as smoke spews from under the hood.

A tow truck takes the car to a mechanic who reveals that the car is nearly totaled, and it's going to take a lot of time and money to get it fixed. Let's say, for the sake of this example, he cannot dump, exchange, or sell the car. He has to bite the bullet and fix it.

How would he go about doing that? First, find a mechanic that can do the job. Second, get the damaged parts repaired. And then, for Pete's sake, drive better! That last part—learning how to drive better—is *exactly* what has to be done next to rid yourself of back and neck pain.

The Problem

Let's go back to the beginning. Remember the pathway to pain starts in one of two ways. Either a) *Something Bad Happens To You* or b) *You Do Something Wrong.* We have no control over the former, and it's incredibly rare. The latter, however, is completely within our influence and is extremely common.

When you use your back and neck incorrectly, Buckling Points are created—that's the start of The Vicious Cycle. Remember, the occasional mistake in using your back and neck won't do you any harm. Your spine has the ability to "recover." It's only when that mistake goes uncorrected and repeated that the Vicious Cycle takes off. Therein lies the final component to The Solution: The mistakes you're making are hurting you, and they have to be stopped. Otherwise, you will be forever caught in the Vicious Cycle, and getting pain-free will never be an option.

The final component for The Solution is to stop making mistakes, and start using your back and neck correctly. Once you start to do this, the rate of Buckling Point creation in your spine gets reduced drastically. This allows your muscles more time to recoup between mistakes, making the Tipping Point harder to cross. Mechanoreception gets maximized, and nociception minimized, which helps your nervous system function optimally. Lastly, the joints move more normally, which helps preserve your cartilage. All in all, becoming "anti-Buckling Point" in all your movements is the only way to turn off the faucet.

How do you do this? Hire a professional back and neck trainer. She or he will be able to identify what you're doing wrong in your day-to-day life, and then teach you how to correct it. For example, this person will be able to figure out if your lower back pain is coming from your sitting posture at work or your lifting mechanics at home. They will be able to determine if your neck pain is coming from how you stand, hold your child, or drive your car. Their job is to train you on how to use your back and neck better so that you don't keep creating Buckling Points. This type of learning intervention goes by many names including "education" "back school," and "cognitive therapy", but the intent is the same: to give you the know-how necessary to use your back and neck correctly.

Think of it this way…

Imagine being dropped off in the middle of the Amazon rainforest. You have no food or water and no way to communicate with the outside world. What gives you the best chance of staying alive: To rely on your own survival skills or have a guide who has already taken thousands of people out? The answer is obvious!

Research Highlights

Studies show that simply learning how you use your back and neck better provides a pretty good amount of relief, even if you do nothing else.[38-45] In fact, there's evidence that shows that "back school" can be as effective as spinal exercise.[46] This is probably because if you're using your back and neck better, it means that you're activating your deep Stabilizers more often.

Let's be clear: learning how to use your spine better, and then implementing those changes, is vital. However, if you've crossed the Tipping Point, using your spine better is not enough. The dysfunctional muscles, nerves, and joints feed off each other, and have to be addressed individually with treatment targeted directly at them to become functional again and reverse the Vicious Cycle. As we've found throughout this section, it's not the ingredients that make a pie delicious—it's how you combine the ingredients that determine whether the pie is worthy of the dinner table or a trashcan.

For Best Results, Use as Directed

- **The advice must be custom-tailored.** It's been found that the most successful outcomes result not only from being taught improved body mechanics and lifting techniques, but also having someone show you how to apply this newfound knowledge to *your* life—your job, your activity level, your age, your body type, etc. In order to turn off *your* specific faucet, whatever that may be, it has to be done in a way that is unique to you. Yes, you can get a suit jacket from a discount store, and it'll probably look and feel good enough, but let's be honest, good enough isn't really good enough. If you want to look and feel your best, your jacket should be custom-tailored, and so should your back and neck advice.
- **Roll up your sleeves.** Don't go someplace where you sit and listen to a teacher and later try to remember what you've learned. That doesn't cut it. You must be involved in the process, and the process must involve you. Knowledge without action is useless.
- **Using your spine better is different from spinal exercises.** I can't tell you how many times a patient has come to me frustrated, saying something like, "I've been doing the exercises, but I'm still getting pain in my back!" I'll ask,

"Well, when did the pain start to worsen again?"

They answer with, "After I was loading wood in the trailer," or something to that effect.

"Could you show me how you were lifting?" I ask. Then I'll see their back contort as they pretend to pick something off the ground.

"Well, I think I know your problem. You would do well to remember that spinal exercises strengthen your Stabilizers so that your joints can handle more mistakes, but they *don't* make them impervious."

- **Never trust a skinny chef.** Not too long ago one of my patients came in for treatment with an obvious chip on his shoulder. I asked what the problem was since normally he's a happy-go-lucky guy. At his annual checkup, his medical doctor told him to lose weight. He then turned to me and scoffed "And he's fatter than I am!"

  The persons whose advice you seek must practice what they preach. If you have better posture than they do, they're not the trainer for you.
- **Lean on me.** Time after time I've worked with athletes and self-proclaimed health "gurus" who thought they knew it all, but couldn't pass the simplest of proper-usage tests. You may think you have a pretty good grasp on this stuff, but the truth is unless you've had professional grade training, you don't. Accept that you're going to need some help. Besides, I bet you don't have the time, interest, or money to spend the next ten years of your life going back to school and learning about pain relief, biology, chemistry, and human biomechanics. By finding an expert and learning

from them, you can obtain a decade's worth of schooling and probably decades' worth of real-world practice in a short amount of time.

- **Seeking a long-term relationship.** How long do you see a dentist? If you want a healthy, bright, pain-free smile, and to avoid tooth decays and root canals, you'll want to see a dentist periodically for your entire life. Chances are you've already accepted this as a fact. It is the same with your back-and-neck professional-grade trainer. Different seasons of life require different skills. Using your back and neck correctly as a teenager requires a different set of skills than in your twilight years and this "trainer" will serve as your guide through those years.

Where do you find a professional back and neck trainer?

Your best chance of getting pain-free does not rest in the arms of medically trained doctors or surgeons. It does not rest in magic potions, lotions, or pills. Nor does it rest in your average chiropractor, physical therapist, massage therapist, or osteopath. It rests in finding a non-drug, non-surgical, professionally trained expert. You're probably not too happy to read that these experts are hard to find. I personally know of only a handful of doctors who understand all of this, and even fewer with the ability to teach it. Although I can't provide you with a list of names, I can share with you some telltale signs you're in the right place.

1. If they're found in a clinic, gym, or some other professional setting with rehab space.
2. If they have good posture.
3. If they host a special workshop about this type of thing.

4. If, when they assess you (and they should in order to figure out how to apply the rules of correctly using the back and neck to your life), they check things like how you pick up objects, walk, stand, squat, sit, etc.

There's an important note to be made here. Everything that's been described so far are components of The Solution, but not The Solution itself. You've learned a lot, and you've been patient. Now your patience is about to be rewarded as I unveil The Solution. But before we take this next step, I have one last thing to say about learning how to use your spine correctly.

Our Future: Starting Young

I shudder to think of the magnitude of chronic pain our children are facing. Kids these days are simply not told about the importance of their posture and using their spine correctly. And we have no one to blame but ourselves. Most parents, guardians, teachers, and adults are unaware of the spine's impact on health and how to take care of it—how to safely do simple movements like lifting objects off the floor, sitting posture, walking posture, etc. This lack of understanding is directly feeding into the onslaught of chronic pain that Americans are experiencing, and it has to change.

Spinal development happens only over a handful of years, and it's the only time when children are developing habits that will last for the rest of their life. What if during that period we taught them how to use their back and neck correctly? What if they were taught how to sit properly, stand properly, and get up from a seated position properly? What if we ensured that, during this phase in their life, that their back and neck created as few Buckling Points as possible? Then, if a Buckling Point was created, it was corrected immediately? If we did *that* back and neck pain could be all but eradicated.

Indeed, starting with kids is an important part of getting out of this chronic pain and mess we're in. The fact that this isn't happening is a problem, but an even-bigger problem is that it doesn't seem to be on anybody's radar.

If you have kids and you're reading this, I hope you teach them the importance of maintaining a healthy spine with the same intent as you do with brushing their teeth, taking a bath, and applying themselves in school. Because protecting your kids' spines when they're young, will ensure that their spine protects them when they're old.

Chapter 28

The Solution: All Together Now

The whole is greater than the sum of its parts.
—Aristotle, philosopher

Imagine a banana split. What makes it so delicious? Is it the soft-serve ice cream? The perfectly ripened banana? The crunchiness of the nuts? Or maybe it's the mouth-watering hot fudge? No, we can't attribute the deliciousness to any single component because it's when they're combined that the real magic happens.

One Is the Loneliest Number That You'll Ever Do

Consider what you've learned so far. Addressing each part of the Vicious Cycle individually, through adjustments, exercise, hands-on muscle therapy, and training, will get you some pretty good results. The research is clear—doing just one of those is better than doing none of those. If you had to choose only one, the adjustments are proven to be superior.

"Pretty good" results, if you ask me, are pretty lame. I think if you have been suffering from chronic back and neck pain, you'd

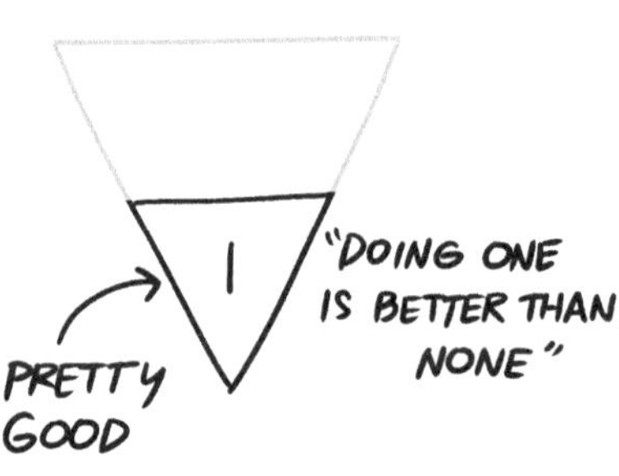

agree. You'd agree if you have tried some of these and you're still in pain. You'd agree if you have watched a loved one turn into a shell of her former selves because of pain. If you've dealt with any type of ongoing, non-resolving pain, you'd agree *that pretty good isn't good enough.*

Two for Your Health

Besides, I didn't write this book for people to get "pretty good," I wrote this book for people to be able to be the best they can be—to be able to do what they want, when they want, and how they want. So, I asked myself, "What if, like the banana split, we were to start combining these interventions? Then what?" This is where it gets exciting.

The research sticks out like a sore thumb: combining any two of those interventions is better than any single one alone. This makes sense. The more of the Vicious Cycle you address, the better. Spinal exercises with massage is better than either one alone. Spinal adjusting, when combined with exercise or education, is also better than any of those alone. Literally, any two you can think of has been proven better than one,[53,18,46,54,38,50] and that's good.

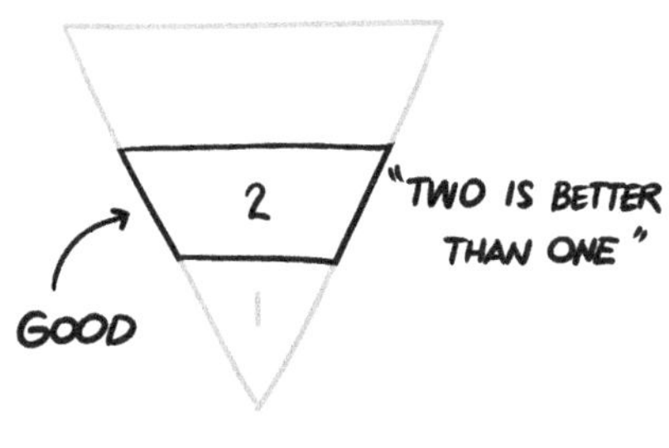

Three's Company

It makes sense that addressing more of the Vicious Cycle would get things better, but is there proof that combining three of those interventions is better than two?

If there is evidence of this, then there is a definite trend that addressing more of the parts that go wrong during the Vicious Cycle will get you better results. One day, in between seeing patients, I was leisurely reading through an 800+ page report on non-invasive treatment of pain (yes, I *am* that obsessive). Then it hit me like a ton of bricks. The clouds opened, a ray of light shone on me, I stood up, and shouted, "Eureka!"

First, I ran across a study that showed that exercise, massage, and education was effective at relieving low back pain.[56] This is important because it proves that combining these three didn't overload the body but instead helped people get better, but it didn't answer the question, "Does combining three of those interventions get people better than two?"

Then, I read how exercise, massage, and education was proven to be more effective than exercise and education alone.[55] This means each individual intervention contributes to relieving pain in its own unique way and if you take a piece away, the results suffer. But what this study was lacking was any information on the keystone treatment: spinal adjustments.

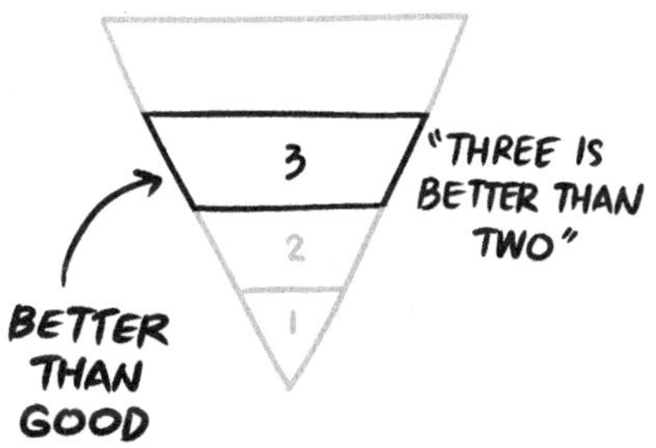

Then, I saw it. Education, exercise, AND adjustments had an even better outcome in relieving pain.[52]

Not only that, combining those three also improved people's general health, faulty back pain beliefs (aka pain myths), and disability. This showed that combining any three of those interventions provided more relief than combining two.

This is really significant because now there's a trend.

Putting Your Best Foot Four-ward

A car has four bad tires. If you do anything less than replace all four, you still have a problem, right? I think you see what's coming. Joint dysfunction must be fixed, Stabilizers must be strengthened, Movers must be remodeled, and Buckling Points must be stopped.

What's the *best* way to do this?

Spinal Adjusting and Spinal Exercises +
Hands-on Muscle Therapy + Training =
The Best Chance for Maximum Relief

That's The Solution, ladies and gentlemen. Plain and simple. *That* is the best way to get the back and neck out of pain. And *that* is what will harness the powerful nerve connection between your muscles, joints, and brain, and bring your back and neck to the ***Turning Point***—where the momentum from breaking down is shifted to the momentum of building up. From dysfunction to function. From destruction to healing. From pathologically

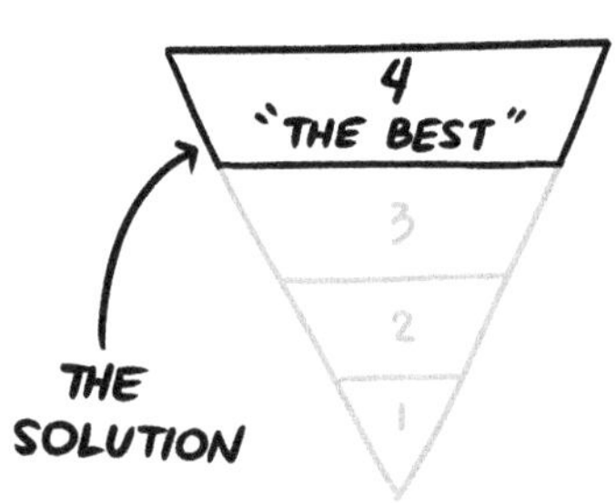

being protected to healthily expressing potential. From pain-full-ness to pain-free-ness. And all because the combination of those four things correct the three unique elements of the spine—the nerves, muscles, and joints—making your back and neck as healthy as possible.

Things to Remember:

1. **A back and neck that is as pain-free as possible is one that is as healthy as possible.** Any effective intervention aims at accomplishing this task.
2. **The most effective way to correct a dysfunctional spinal joint is through spinal adjustments.** The science is clear: adjustments are the gold standard for this type of problem. If you don't fix the joints, the muscles will stay bad.
3. **The most effective way to strengthen the deep Stabilizers is spinal exercises.** Anything short of this simply will not get the job done. Remember, practice does not make prefect. Only perfect practice makes perfect.
4. **The most effective way to get rid of scar tissue and tightness in the superficial Movers is through hands-on muscle therapy.** Sometimes you'll have to get your hands dirty to get the job done. That's the case for ridding scar tissue-induced knots in your muscles, and stimulating the formation of longer and stronger muscles.
5. **Find an expert to help you identify what you're doing wrong, and help you fix it.** There's no way to get around it. You'll need someone else's help if you're to ever get free of pain. This person will be your partner in getting you

better, but remember, you had a large role getting into this mess (unless *Something Bad Happened To You*), and you'll have a large role getting out of this mess.

6. **The most effective way to get your back and neck out of pain is to combine the adjustments with exercise, hands-on muscle therapy, and training.**

Chapter 29

How Long Is This Going to Take?

Time heals all wounds.—Unknown

I wish I could say that The Solution works like a light switch: you flip it on, and you're instantly pain-free. But that's not how it works. The Vicious Cycle has built up momentum, and simply can't be stopped on a dime. Like a locomotive going "full steam ahead," it must be slowed–*then* stopped. Once that's been accomplished, then and only then, is it possible to shift that momentum.

All of this takes time. That's the bad news.

The good news is that the amount of time it takes has been proven through research.

Phase 1: The Recovery/Inflammatory Phase

It's during this phase where the Vicious Cycle slows, stops, and you hit a Turning Point—where your back and neck start healing up rather than continuing to break down. This is a big deal and a big step in the right direction of being pain-free.

However, it doesn't guarantee you start to feel better. It may surprise you to learn that you might actually feel worse as you go through this phase. Why? Because your back and neck has sensitized nerves, damaged joints, atrophied and scar tissue-ridden muscles, and the treatment is going to spark some inflammation. Be warned: while applying The Solution and getting your back and neck into this phase is really good for you, you can certainly feel worse during it.

Then again, you might not. Some people feel the same, and others do feel better. It all depends on the condition of *your* back and neck.

This phase can take as little as three days, or quite often between eight to twelve weeks—or much longer.[57,58,59]

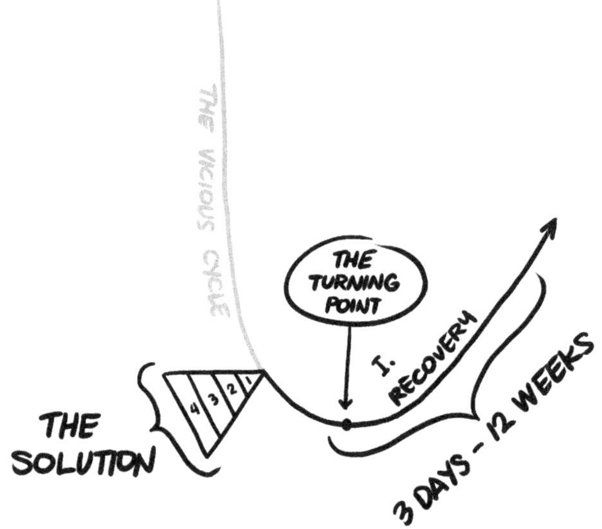

The fastest way to get you through this phase is with structured and frequent care. Some people need to start with daily treatments.[60,61] Others could get by with treatment two to three times a week. It all depends on *your* back and neck, *your* history, and *your* activity level.

Phase 2: Repair and Remodeling

After the Recovery/Inflammation Phase, your body enters into Phase 2: Repair and Remodeling.

During the **Repair** phase, muscles are rebuilt, ligaments are restructured, resistance returns to the nerves, and sometimes discs are regenerated—all, to the degree that the permanent pathological changes allow. The thing is, there's a problem with all of the new tissue being laid down: it's immature, fresh, and weak, which means that there is a risk that the dysfunction and damage could come back. The body, with its intelligence, does something about this. It moves into the next phase

During the **Remodeling** portion of this phase, the "newbie" tissue starts to earn its keep. Amazingly, as the newer tissues get stretched and strained with use, they begin to get stronger.

The important bit to remember is that during this phase, you'll probably start to feel better, but you're not healed yet and shouldn't act like you are. If your house caught on fire (don't worry; everything that is near and dear to you was saved), and you were in the process of rebuilding, would you live in the house while you put up the scaffolding and erected its frame? No. Should you start to refurnish the living room before the floors are put in? No, of course not. You don't start living in the house until the repairs are finished, right? Same rule of thought applies to your back and neck during this phase in the healing process. You don't start "living" in your back and neck until the repairs are finished.

Outside of the direct supervision of The Solution expert, you need to be incredibly careful of your postures and movements, and put as little undue stress on your back and neck as possible. Inside of the Solution expert's clinic, your care is still frequent and structured in order to achieve full range of motion and maintain it through this phase.

For your body this means that:

- Your spinal adjustments and hands-on muscle therapy are still happening pretty close to two to three times a week.
- Your deep Stabilizers are strengthened, smartened, and taught to have endurance through daily exercising, stretching, and mobilizing.

For sure, this is a demanding schedule, but it is the best protocol for getting pain-free. The good news is that during this phase, the frequency of treatment can start getting less. The keys for decreased frequency are that you:

- Prove you have stopped doing the "*Something Wrong*," and know how to do it right.
- Pass a baseline muscle coordination, strength, and endurance test.
- Demonstrate competency in performing a home exercise program.
- Have maintained an as-full-as possible range of motion for a minimum of ninety days.

To start functioning optimally and maximize pain relief, all of these things must be present for the duration of the Repair phase: one to six months[57,59,62].

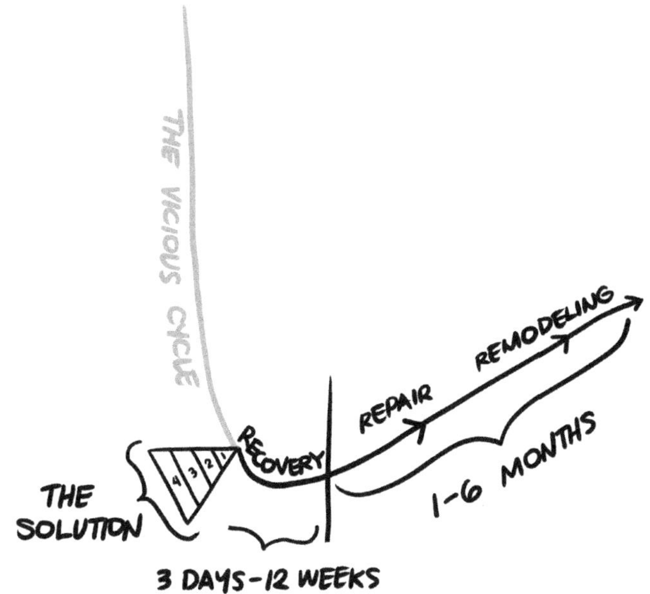

Phase 3: Stabilization

New tissue has been laid down. Muscles are rebuilt stronger, longer, and smarter than before. Cartilage is resilient and squishy vs. degenerated and decaying. The motion of your spine is as full as possible, and your individual spinal segments are moving as best they can. This gives your brain optimal input, and it's making sure that your back and neck are functioning optimally. All of this allows you to be as close to pain-free as possible because all of the things that were causing your pain are made anew, right? Wrong! What? How can that be? You might ask, "I've already come this far, so how can I not be completely out of pain?"

It's because *new* tissue has been laid down, like a fresh scab. Sure, it's there, covering up the cut, stopping it from getting worse—the Repair Phase—heck, that scab can toughen up—the

Remodeling Phase—but it's still a scab, and if you brush it against something, what happens to it? It opens up again.

After Phase 1 and Phase 2, your back and neck enters into Phase 3: Stabilization. During this phase, the new changes get cemented into place. Through a process of trial and error and tears and repairs, the body gets tough and resilient. Not only the muscle and joints, mind you, but most importantly, the nerves. Your brain forms new neurons, learns new posture and movement habits so that if you do something incorrectly again, or something bad happens to you, and a Buckling Point is created, your back and neck does not hit the Tipping Point quite so easily. If it does, the spine won't go back to its *old mold.* Not a chance. Your brain, because it's been retrained, actually pushes the body to heal in the *new mold...* a more *pain-free mold...* a *"live-life-the-way-you want-to" mold.*

This phase is when the scab has turned back into skin. And that's not all. This is typically when you can be released with your own, custom-tailored, home-care program. This should involve a unique combination of specific exercises, mobilizations, stretches, non-drug pain relief techniques, and dietary guidelines designed for you. Also, your spinal adjustment frequency can be reduced to once or twice every two to four weeks.[63,64] This level of support needs to be maintained anywhere from one to two years after the completion of the Repair Phase[65,57,59,66] in order for you to get pain-free. During this phase, you will be thrilled to feel the best you have through the whole healing process. Remember: *your spine is not your tongue.* The tongue, because of all the blood that's in it, heals ridiculously fast. The spine is literally the opposite because tissues like deep spine cartilage, nerves, ligaments, etc. have a very scant blood supply.

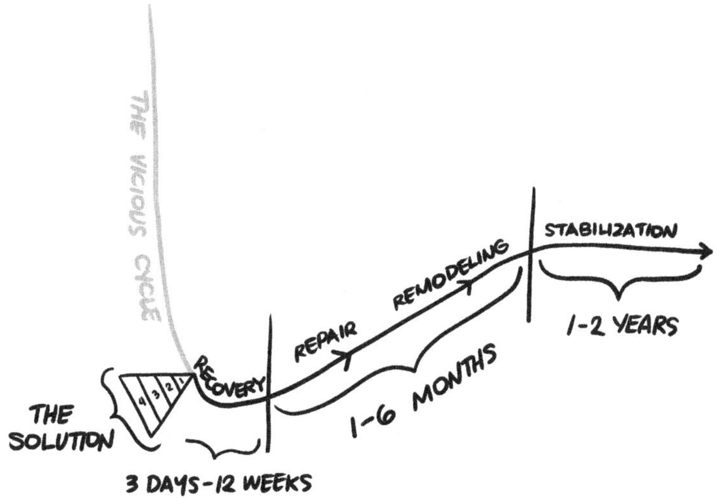

Final Thought

Hippocrates, the father of medicine, said that *"Healing is a matter of opportunity and time."* By implementing The Solution, you're giving the body the opportunity to get pain free. All that's left is time.

For Best Results, Use as Directed

- **Repetition is the mother of learning.** At the beginning of this journey to a pain-free life, you and your spine are going to be in a tug-of-war battle. Your muscles and nerves are so accustomed to being weak and contracted that they are ready to drag the joints right back to the way they were after your first treatments. Over time, though, the tissues will begin to change, and eventually they will help your joints stay moving. It takes repetition—a lot of it—and although the schedule laid out is pretty demanding, if you truly want to get pain-free, this is absolutely the best protocol.

- **The three-to-four visit myth.** I've had patients tell me they've heard that "If you're not feeling better in three or four visits, it's not going to work." Not only is that statement unscientific and not based on evidence, it's just plain stupid. How could a condition that has taken months, or quite probably years, to develop, heal within three to four visits over a week or two? It doesn't make sense. Plus, it's physiologically impossible. This is simply a myth propagated by people who don't know what they're talking about.

  Here's the truth: How long it takes you to get out of pain depends on how long you've been in pain, and how far down the Vicious Cycle your back and neck have gone. If you have experienced the pain for three months or less, you'll have a relatively quick turnaround. If the pain has been bothering you for longer than three months, you're in for a considerably longer haul. One study went as far as to say that "Increased function and reduction of pain may not occur for 12 weeks."[67] Keep that in mind as you set off on the road to a pain-free destination.
- **Just do it.** During all of these phases, while it's important to be mindful of what you're doing, you can't stop "doing." Keep doing your regular daily activities, especially the ones that you want to do, whether that's gardening, playing with the kids, golfing, or traveling. It's only by *doing* that your back and neck learns what it needs to do in order for you to *keep doing.*
- **Stable but not fixed.** Once you've completed the Stabilization Phase you'll be declared *stable*, but not *fixed.* Nothing in your body is ever fixed once and then is good to go

forever. Although you've been through all of this, if you start doing things wrong again, your back and neck will become dysfunctional again, and then it's back into the Vicious Cycle.

- **Get your oil changed frequently.** It's good to get the back and neck stable again (who wants to be unstable?), but it's much better to keep it that way—like getting your car's oil changed frequently after you've had the engine fixed. For your spine, that means you should keep doing exercises, keep stretching, keep mobilizing, and keep your diet clean. It also means getting your back and neck checked periodically to ensure that the areas that have been permanently damaged are staying in check. How often should you do the home care program? Daily, like brushing your teeth. How often should you get your spine checked? Once a week to once every four weeks—your Solution expert will be able to help you with that.
- **Plant a tree today.** Guess what's the most common comment patients make when I tell them about the healing phases and the time it takes? You have almost certainly said the same thing to yourself while reading this chapter. Are you ready? Here it is: "Gee-whiz! I don't have time for that!" I agree that's probably true. It is a major time commitment. I also know if you're reading this, you're probably in pain or someone you know is in pain. Mother Nature has certain requirements that must be met in order to heal. And in learning the amount of time it takes to complete the journey to become pain-free, I hope you've realized two things. First, if you're not in pain, keep yourself that way

The best time to plant a tree was twenty years ago, the next best time is now.

by installing The Solution as a part of your life. Second, remember this saying: "The best time to plant a tree was twenty years ago, the next best time is now."

Chapter 30

The Big Picture

Sometimes you've got to take a big step back to see the full picture.—Anonymous

Take a moment and let this image digest in your mind.

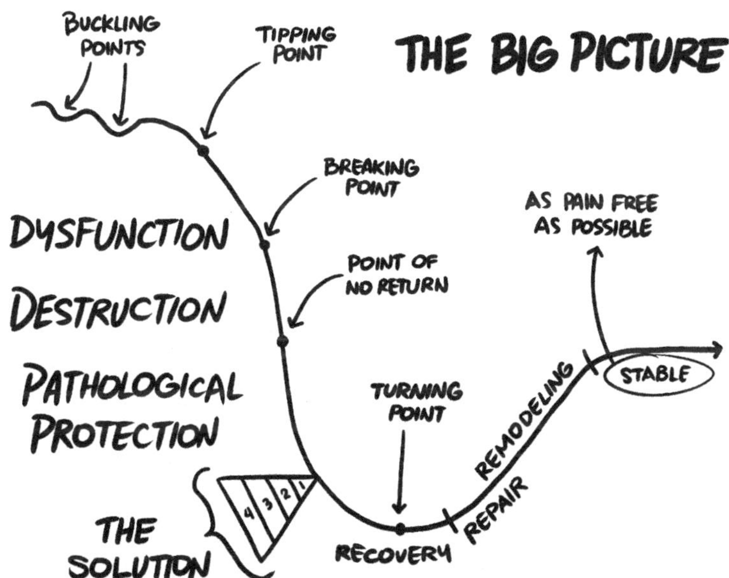

If there's anything that doesn't look familiar, you've missed something, and it's well worth your time going back and figuring it out. On the other hand, if you understand what you're seeing, you can sleep well tonight knowing that you understand more about back and neck pain than your average Joe and probably more than most doctors. Nice work!

We've come a long way, you and me, and now it's time to take one last step.

SECTION 6

The Last Step: Take Action

To be is to do. —Immanuel Kant

Chapter 31

Oh, Henry!

The results you achieve will be in direct proportion to the effort you apply
—Denis Waitley, author, speaker, productivity consultant

After my patient, Henry, had told me that his lower back pain was interfering with his relationship with his kids, he sat there with a somewhat embarrassed look. I put down my clipboard and pen, and met his gaze.

"Henry, I want to make sure you and I are on the same page. What specific result are you looking for by being here?"

His head cocked to the side thoughtfully. "I know my pain will probably never go away completely, but I want less of it. I want my back to get good enough that the kids tire out before I do. I want to be the father I think they deserve." He had certainty in his voice, like a man on a mission.

Nodding in understanding, I said, "I'm going to make a promise to you, Henry. If I examine you and truly find I cannot get you that result, I'll tell you. If I can, I'll tell you that, too. Does that sound fair?"

He nodded in agreement, though he didn't say much more. He was still somewhat withdrawn and hesitant.

The rest of Henry's visit was full of diagnostic questions, a physical examination, orthopedic testing, and x-ray images. It became apparent that, while Henry was physically fit, his lower back was weak and he was already very deep into the Vicious Cycle.

As the visit came to a close, I placed my trusty clipboard on the counter and put my pen in its rightful place behind my ear. "I think it would be best if we didn't rush into treatment. I feel good about getting the results you want, but I want to take the time to review my findings, confirm them, and then develop an actionable plan.

As a child, I remember standing next to my grandfather, a farmer and carpenter, as he stood at his workbench.

"Why do you keep marking that same piece of wood, Grandpa?" I had asked.

I still remember the way he chuckled and patted my head. "Benjamin," he'd said with his thick Norwegian accent, "Measure twice and cut once."

I've carried that with me always, applying it to my life in other ways. That was exactly what I planned to do for Henry.

Henry returned the next day. He wasn't what I'd call *chipper* to be in my office again, but he knew that I wanted to help him. So instead of grunts and scowling, I had something closer to complete sentences and attentiveness. We were making progress.

"I have good news for you, Henry," I said, this time firming up my grip as my hand entered into the trash compactor known as Henry's handshake. "I believe I can help you eliminate this pain and get you to the point where you can play with your boys again."

At that, he smiled the first I smile I had seen from him since we'd met. For the next half-hour, I explained the problem with his lower back and went over the treatment details, telling him he needed specific spinal adjustments, therapeutic exercises, and deep, hands-on muscle therapy.

"Here's the deal, though," I began, a note of warning in my tone, "You may want to prepare yourself for a long haul. It could take anywhere from four to six months to really get your lower back under control."

He hesitated, heaving a long sigh as he mulled over the statement. Not only would it require a huge time commitment from him, but he knew his insurance coverage was limited. At last, he replied, "I wanna do this, doc. I *need* to."

It took at least four weeks before we saw any kind of improvement. In fact, his entire course of care was riddled with flare-ups and setbacks. Little by little, however, we made progress.

By the end of his treatment, we'd developed a good relationship, and Henry wasn't the same intimidating, hesitant person he had been when he'd first arrived. He was someone who had dedicated himself to doing what it takes to eliminate chronic back pain—an inspiring transformation to observe.

At last, I performed a final reexamination of his lower back to assess its stability. We discussed his overall improvement: his spinal range-of-motion had increased by over fifty percent; he passed all of the stress tests for his lower back Stabilizers; and he could demonstrate how to lift things without creating Buckling Points.

"You're stable, Henry!"

He looked at me blankly, which threw me off. I was excited about his improvements, but he was oddly quiet.

Then, in typical Henry fashion, short and to-the-point, he said, "Doc, I really don't care about all that." I felt my throat constrict and I swallowed hard. After a moment, he smiled as he said, "All I care about is how I felt last night and today."

"And how's that?"

"When my boys asked me to wrestle, I didn't give it a second thought. I got down on the floor and showed them who's boss," he said with pride. "And here's the best part: I didn't hurt then, and I don't hurt now."

Chapter 32

Apply The Solution

Talk doesn't boil the rice.—Dr. Joseph Sweere, chiropractor, professor at Northwestern Health Science University

At this point, you understand that the back and neck have to go through quite a few steps in order for pain to develop. You also understand that eliminating pain, especially if it's chronic or reoccurring, can take a few steps as well. You've learned the truth behind the most dangerous myths concerning back and neck pain, and have gone through the depths of the Vicious Cycle. You've also learned the most commonsense and evidence-based Solution to back and neck pain. And now you're there, wherever that is, with this book in your hands.

Do you hear that?

That's the sound of your life calling you to take the last step: Apply The Solution, eliminate your back and neck pain, and get your life back.

Good luck and God Speed.

Chapter 33

The Daily 5

An apple a day keeps the doctor away.—Anonymous

When I first discovered the research showing how many people are dealing with pain, I had to ask myself, why? Why are episodes of pain so frequent? Why will nearly everyone experience some back and neck pain?

I came to realize that most people don't know how to use their back and neck properly. Think about it. Aren't we told the importance of washing our hands every flu season? Aren't we all taught in school how to take care of our teeth? "Brush and floss, or else your teeth will rot and fall out." However, when are we taught the importance of using our spine correctly? When are we told of the rotten consequences that come with the misuse? Rarely, if ever.

To address this, as a bonus, I'm going to show you five daily habits that, if you actually develop them, will take a great deal of stress off your spine. These "The Daily 5" are at the foundation of any training designed to prevent Buckling Points. That being said, it's important for you to know that these five, while a great step in the right direction, are just that…a step. On their own, they will not get you to your final destination—being pain-free, but you should already know that if you've made it this far.

The Daily 5

1. **Chin Tuck: Your new, annoying, daily habit.**
2. **Hip Hinge: The single most important maneuver that you forgot you knew.**
3. **Belly Breathing: Why "tucking in your gut" is not okay.**
4. **Spine Stretch: Like brushing your teeth, but for your back and neck.**
5. **Nutrition: You feel what you eat!**

The Daily 5 are actually very simple. And they focus around one key point: Never bend your spine. In his book, *Becoming a Supple Leopard*, Kelly Starrett, Doctor of Physical Therapy and all around genius, states, "The majority of human movements require you to move through a full range-of-motion without defaulting into a broken spinal position." (Author paraphrase)

What is a "broken spinal position?" It is simply another phrase for a Buckling Point, which most commonly occur when, instead of curving, your spine becomes bent.

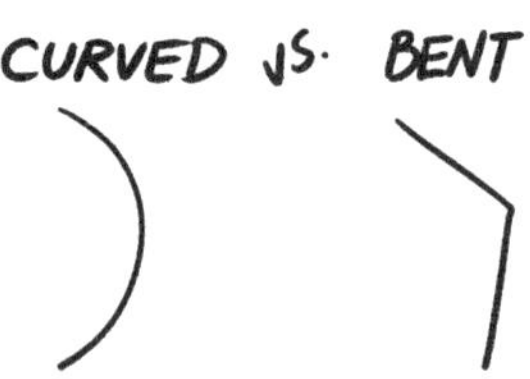

Like a guy lying on a bed of a thousand nails, when the spine is curved the stress gets spread out across multiple spots. What happens if you remove all the nails except one and have the guy lie on it? What will you have? That's right, a human shish kabob. This is because all of the stress has now focused on a single spot and that damages the body. That's exactly what happens to the back and neck when the spine is bent. All of the stress gets focused on one joint and it gets damaged.

Dr. Starrett also says, "If you see flexion or extension (forward bent or backward bent) anywhere in the spine, it's an error." That's exactly what needs to be avoided. Here's how to do it.

1. Chin Tuck: Your new, annoying, daily habit.

When was the last time you considered the position of your head? Like where it's sitting in relation to your back and neck? Probably not until you finished that sentence. That's a problem.

When I was a teenager, I coached our local diving team. For the divers who wanted to do a front flip, we would teach them one concept: "Where the head goes, the body follows." The moment they leapt off the board, they would quickly flex their head downward. The momentum of that movement would carry them into a flipping motion. We taught a lot of kids to do flips like this—to the dismay of many mothers.

The position of your head is important because your head is heavy. It's at least 10–15 pounds, and it sits on top of a mostly unsupported part of your spine, your neck. The mid back is reinforced by ribs and the abdominal contents. The low back is supported by the pelvis, quite a bit of muscle, and more organs. But your neck is left to fend for itself. Therein lies a potential problem.

If you don't position your head correctly, you'll constantly create Buckling Points in your neck.

Here's an example. In my reception area, we have a coffee bar where patients can enjoy a warm drink. One day, I walked out into the reception area as a young woman was finishing her hot chocolate. I watched in horror as she bent her neck back and brought her chin up to take a drink. It looked like this:

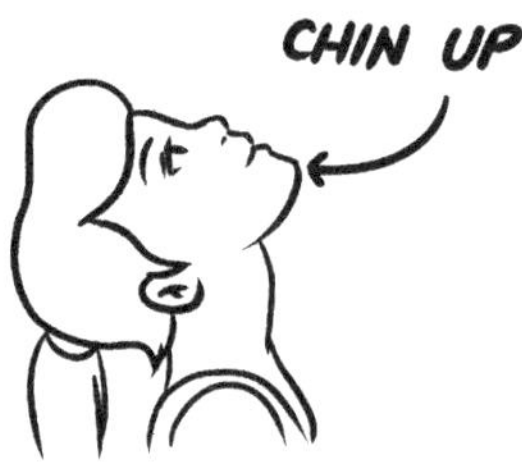

You might be thinking, "You're seriously going to tell me that the way I've been drinking is wrong. Get a life, man." But stick with me for a second. If you had X-ray vision and could see inside of her neck, this is what you'd see.

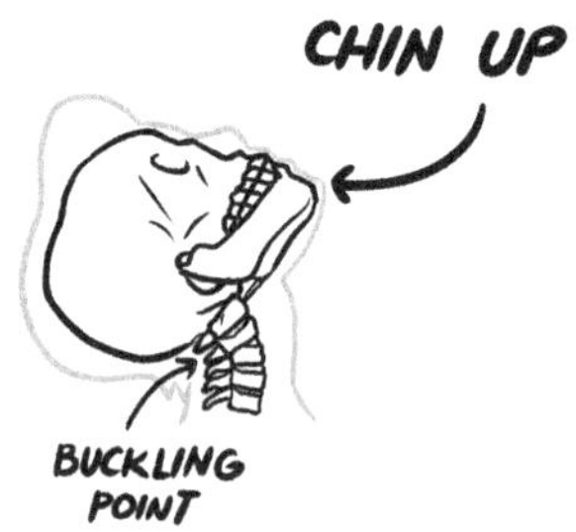

Notice the Buckling Point in the middle of the neck. That's a bend, a broken spinal position. Get this. Later that evening, I was having dinner with a close friend, his wife, and their adorable two-year-old daughter. I watched this toddler pick up her cup and take a drink from it. This time, instead of horror, I watched in amazement. First, she grasped the cup in both hands and brought it to her lips. Then she tucked her chin and extended her entire upper body. This caused her neck and upper back to curve, allowing her spine to completely avoid creating a Buckling Point.

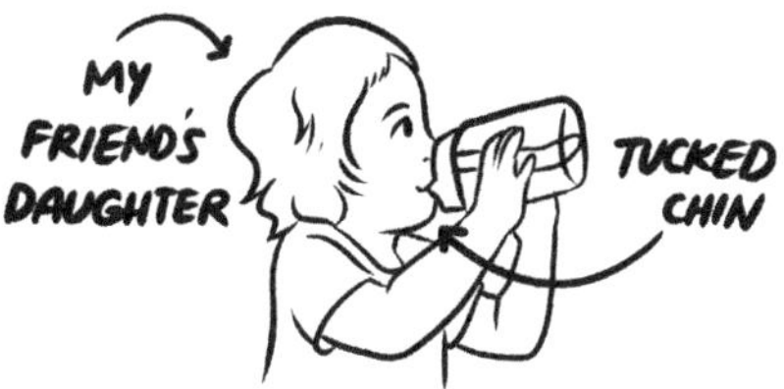

Using your X-ray vision again, you would see that she didn't bend her neck at all. Instead, she curved it.

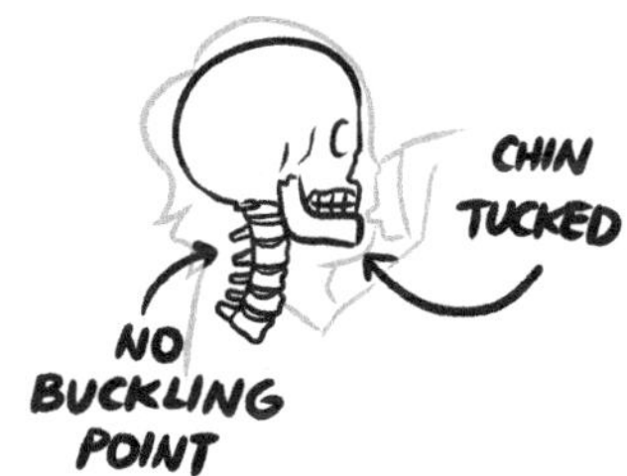

In order to curve your neck and not bend it, you'll need to master a special move that gives you the ability to control the position of your head: The Chin Tuck.

Imagine you have a string tied to the top of your head, and it's being pulled up and back. How would your head and neck move?

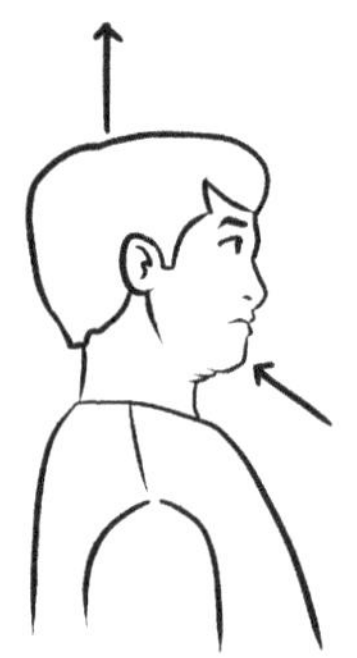

When you move like this, it's as if you're giving yourself a double chin, but in doing so, you optimize your neck's curve, and effectively avoid bending it. Before you take a drink of water, bench press, sit and work at the computer, or bring a spoonful of soup to your mouth, first, set your Chin Tuck. It should become your new but annoying daily habit. You'll know you're doing it right when friends and family look at you and ask, "What in the world are you doing with your head?"

Going back to the adorable two-year-old, what astounded me the most about her correct use of her back and neck to do something as simple as taking a drink—was that *she simply did it.* She didn't watch a YouTube video or read this book. She didn't have special instruction or attend a weekend seminar. *She just did it.* It must've felt right. On a different occasion, I watched her squat to pick up a toy from the ground. She did that in perfect form, too. Later, I observed my own nieces doing the same thing. Never did I see them take a drink of water or pick something up with a bent spine. It was always a nice Chin Tuck or squat—the back staying straight, the butt sticking out, so that bending occurs at the hips.

This drove me crazy. How can these children, who can't go to the bathroom by themselves have nearly perfect movement and posture?

Then like a lightning bolt, the answer struck me: Our back and neck comes preprogrammed for proper use. That's the default setting of our bodies. But when they get forced into the Vicious Cycle, it all gets lost. What that tells us is if we do something incorrectly long enough, before long we will be forced to keep doing that thing incorrectly. As we all know, the more mistakes we make with the back and neck, the more likely you're going to be in pain.

Now, on to the next one.

2. Hip Hinge: The single most important maneuver that you forgot you knew.

The next installment to undo the bad programming focuses on low back and hips. Dr. Eric Goodman and Peter Park, in their amazing book, *Foundation*, note that, "Bending from the waist distorts the natural curves of the spinal column. The curve of the spinal column should be *retained* while bending forward." (author paraphrase)

When you bend from your waist, you are actually bending your low back, thus creating a Buckling Point. That's not good.

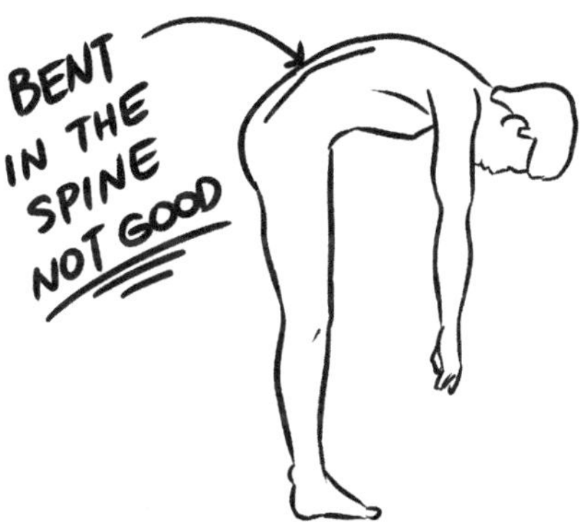

What do you do? Don't bend from the waist—*hinge at the hips.*

By "hinging at the hips," you keep your lower back straight, your butt gets pushed back, and your hips absorb all the force, which is exactly what they're designed to do.

The steps to do this are: stand with your feet shoulder-width apart. Bend your knee slightly. Keep your weight on your heels.

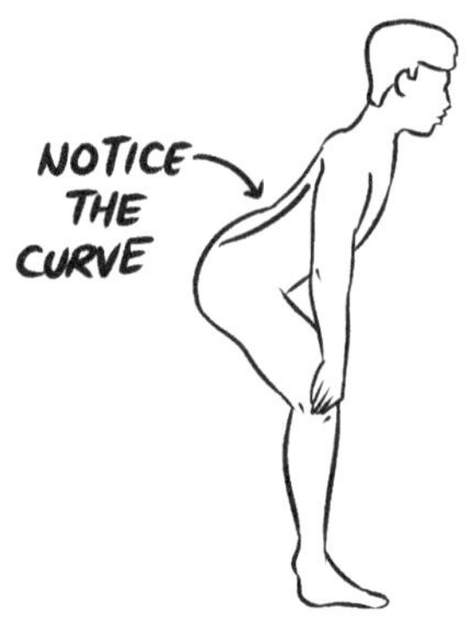

Push your butt back. Now you're in position to hinge at your hips. Now lower yourself.

Like the Chin Tuck, the more you do this, the more natural it'll feel, and the better you'll get. Before you bend forward to pick up the clothes from the floor, golf ball from the hole, or backpack from the ground, be sure to hinge at your hips,

3. Belly Breathing: Why "tucking in your gut" is not okay.

Yoga practitioners have believed for centuries that each person only has so many breaths to take in their lifetime. That's part of the reason why, if you've ever done yoga, you've heard your instructor comment on controlling your breathing. It's believed that if you can control how you breathe, you can control when you take your last breath.

Now, I don't know if that's true, but what I do know is that *how* you breathe is either hurting or helping your chances to be pain-free.

Breathing is one of the most important things for a pain-free back and neck because it involves how you use your diaphragm. Your diaphragm is the muscle that regulates your breathing, and it's there first to expand your lungs to suck in air so that you can stay alive. That's really important. Secondly, because it attaches throughout the middle back, when it is strong and being used correctly, it also helps to stabilize that area—which is the link between your neck and lower back. That's important too. You could do the Chin Tuck all day and Hip Hinge at every opportunity, but if your breathing is off, you'll never be quite as good as you could be. Truth be told, if you don't breathe in the correct manner, you're actually nudging your back and neck closer and closer to the Tipping Point.

Remember the Breathing Test I had you take during the Vicious Cycle? I did this because if your shoulders raise when you breathe in, it means that the superficial Movers have taken over, and the deep Stabilizers of your neck have gone weak—hallmarks of the Dysfunction Phase.

Now, if this is happening every time you take a breath, that dysfunction is being reinforced over and over. Consider how much you actually breathe. You take somewhere around 20,000 breaths per day, and 20,000 is a lot of anything. If you're doing it wrong, it's 20,000 small nudges in the wrong direction, or 20,000 small nudges in the right direction if are you doing it right.

Here's how to ensure you're doing it right:

1. Lie on your back,
2. Put one hand on your chest,
3. Put the other hand on your belly,
4. Take a deep breath in and push out your belly (you should feel your hand rise),
5. Exhale, and you should feel your belly lower, and
6. Do it again.

Remember: Your neck and shoulders shouldn't move at all during this.

By the way, since we've been talking about toddlers and how perfectly they do things, the next time you're near a toddler, look at his stomach as he breathes. Guess what you'll see? When he breathes in, his belly goes out—and that's the key. The trick is to apply this with every breath. You should be doing it when you sit, when you stand, when you go for a run, when you're driving your car, and when you're making supper. The more you do this, the better you'll be for it.

4. Spine Stretch: Like brushing your teeth, but for your back and neck.

Compared to what we already covered, this next one is different. The first three are habits that you need to get used to doing all the time, day in and day out. This next one is something you do once or twice a day.

Because all humans are front heavy, as gravity pulls on us it not only pulls us down, but it also pulls us forward. This wreaks havoc on the spine because this constant pressure compresses your spinal joints. Combining this with sitting and poor lifting mechanics means most of us are headed for a world of hurt, or if you're already in one, headed toward a place where the world hurts more.

The fourth habit is decompressing your spine. The back and neck absolutely love this because it takes pressure off of them. It stretches the muscle, discs, and ligaments, giving them a chance to recover. All in all, decompression to your spine is like a glass of cool water on a hot day.

How do you do it? Tons of gadgets out there all boast they're the best. The most common one is an inversion table—where you hang upside down. While they may have their merits, my educated opinion: they're not the best. They simply don't allow you the range of motion and freedom that you really need. Besides, I've found a cheaper and more effective way to decompress your spine. It's called the **Spine Stretch**. Here's how to do it.

Once you purchase a gym ball, inflate it so that it is firm. Then:

1) Sit on the gym ball,
2) Walk yourself out while leaning back so that your back rests against the ball,
3) Push with your legs, and extend your back over the ball,
4) Keep your head rested fully against the ball—you should not have your head lifted, and
5) Once stable, let your arms extend over your head.

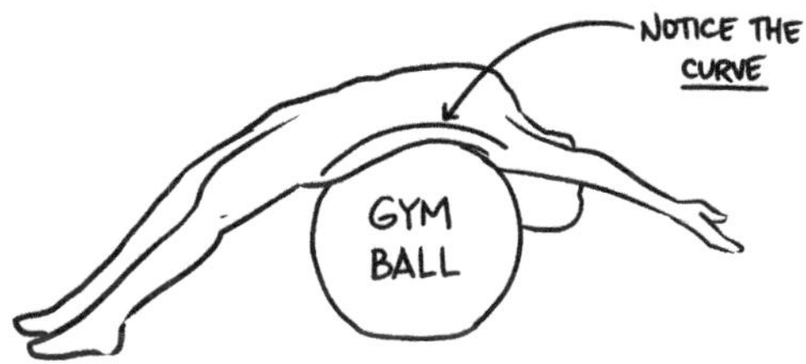

In this position you can quietly lie there and let the decompression and stretch deepen. You could gently rock yourself back and forth—that's good for you because you actively pump new fluids into your spine. You could roll to one side and then the other, stretching out your flanks. The beautiful thing is, once you're in this position, you're in control, and virtually any motion you can do will help decompress your spine. The more you do this, the more your back and neck will like you for it.

5. Nutrition: You feel what you eat!

Every morsel of food that enters your mouth is either moving you closer to pain or farther away. You're either starving inflammation or feeding it. There is no in-between and no foods are neutral. You must be careful what you eat if you're ever to become pain-free.

Here are a few guidelines to follow during your pursuit of pain-free living. Be forewarned, the relationship between diet and pain is fairly complex, enough so that entire books have been dedicated to this topic. What I'm about to divulge is by no means comprehensive, but it is a good place to start.

Foods to avoid: Alcohol, omega-6 cooking oils, dairy products, processed meats, refined grains, white bread, rice, pasta, artificial food additives, aspartame, monosodium glutamate (MSG), sugars, trans fats, and commercially produced meats where the animals are fed grains.

Foods to consume: asparagus, avocado, beets, Brussel sprouts, broccoli, cauliflower, kale, parsnips, spinach, Romaine lettuce, berries, apples, oranges, pears, lemon, cantaloupe, green tea, turkey, chicken, eggs, and salmon.

Omega-3 Fatty Acids: this nutrient is absolutely crucial for the elimination of pain *because it regulates inflammation*. If you have too little Omega-3, your body overproduces inflammation, leading to you to feeling more pain than you should. The problem we face is that our modern diet simply doesn't provide enough of it. This means that unless you've been actively supplementing with Omega-3, you're likely deficient. This stuff is so potent that research shows it is as effective as those dangerous NSAIDs we discussed earlier, and the best part is that they have *none* of their side effects.[68] How much should you take? 370/mg per 40 lbs. per day.

Vitamin D: Like Omega-3s, this is another crucial nutrient for the reduction of pain. Here's a quote directly from the research: "Many patients with Vitamin D deficiency may complain of full, persistent, generalized musculoskeletal aches, pains, and weaknesses, fatigue, fibromyalgia, and chronic fatigue syndrome."[70] How much should you take? About 4000IUs (IU stands for International Units and is simply system of measurement like ounces) per day per day for adults and 1000IUs per day for children.[71]

Proteolytic enzymes: Instead of reaching for the aspirin or ibuprofen bottle after a flare up or injury, reach for this. This supplement counteracts inflammation, slows the formation of scar tissue, and improves blood flow to the site of pain or injury. The best part: it does all this by working *with* your body, and not *overriding* it. This is a must have for anyone who is serious about getting out of pain in the most drug-free way.

These five habits are crucial for you to retrain your back and neck, and keep you out of the Vicious Cycle and pain-free. Remember, knowledge is different than action.

Get to it!

NOTE: When you see (n.d.) listed below, it means (no date)—the publication date is missing.

Selected Sources

Section 1

1. Institute of Medicine, Committee on Advance Pain Research, Care, and Education. (2011). *Relieving pain in America: A blueprint for transforming prevention, care, education and research* (pp. 62) Publication copy. Washington, DC: National Academies Press.
2. *The American Academy of Pain Medicine.* American Academy of Pain Medicine. Accessed September 25, 2016. http://www.painmed.org/PatientCenter/Facts_on_Pain.aspx.

Section 2

1. Almekinders, L. An in vitro investigation into the effects of repetitive motion and nonsteroidal anti-inflammatory medication on human tendon fibroblasts. *American Journal of Sports Medicine,* No. 23 (1995): 119-123.
2. Hauser, Russ A. MD, E.E. Dolan, H.J. Phillips, A.C. Newlin, R.E. Moore, B.A. Woldin.. "Ligament Injury and Healing: A Review of Current Clinical Diagnostics and Therapeutics," *The Open Rehabilitation Journal,* No. 6 (2013): 1-20.
3. Chestnut, J. L. The 14 *Foundational Premises for the Scientific and Philosophical Validation of the Chiropractic Wellness Paradigm*. Victoria, B.C.: Wellness Practice, 2003.

4. Moynihan, R. "Who pays for the pizza? Redefining the relationships between doctors and drug companies," BMJ 326 no. 7400 (2003): 1189-1192. doi:10.1136/bmj.326.7400.1189
5. "Pharmaceutical Research and Development: What Do We Get for All That Money?" *BMJ* 345 (August, 2012). doi: http://dx.doi.org/10.1136/bmj.e4348
6. Mosbergen, D. (n.d.). *Tylenol Overdose Risk Is Staggering; Acetaminophen Safeguards Remain Insufficient*: Report. Retrieved May 23, 2016, from http://www.huffingtonpost.com/2013/09/24/tylenol-overdose_n_3976991.html.
7. William M. Lee, MD (2012). *Opioid-Acetaminophen Combination Products: Should They Be Removed from the Market?* AASLD Clinical Research Single Topic Conference Acetaminophen Poisoning
8. Manthripragada, A. D., E. H. Zhou, M. C. Lovegrove, and M. E. Willy. "Characterization of Acetaminophen Overdose-Related Emergency Department Visits and Hospitalizations in the United States." *Pharmacoeidemiology and Drug Safety* 20, no. 8 (February 3, 2011): 819-26. Accessed November 4, 2016. doi:10.1002/pds.2090.
9. Ganley, Charles, MD, Gerald Dal Pan, MHS, and Bob Rappaport, MD. Department of Health and Human Services, Food and Drugs Administration, Center for Drug Evaluation and Research. (2009). Memorandum: *Background Package for June 29-30, 2009 Meeting*. To: Advisory Committee members, Drug Safety and Risk Management Committee, Anesthetic and Life Support Drugs Advisory Committee and Nonprescription Drugs Advisory Committee.

10. Wolfe, M. M., M.D., D. R. Lichtenstein, M.D., and G. Singh, M.D. (1999). "Gastrointestinal Toxicity of Nonsteroidal Anti-inflammatory Drugs." *New England Journal of Medicine, 1888–1899,* 1999. Retrieved from http://www.drtheo.com/news/NSAIDs.pdf.
11. Emmert, Roberts, Vanessa Delgado Nunes, Sara Buckner, Susan Latchem, Margaret Constanti, Paul Miller, Michael Doherty, et. al. *Paracetamol: Not as Safe as We Thought? A Systematic Literature Review of Observational Studies.* Down loaded from http://ard.bmj.com/ on May 14, 2016—Published by group.bmj.com.
12. Breitner, J C.S., MD, MPH; S J.P.A. Haneuse, PhD, R Walker, MS, S Dublin, MD, PhD, P K. Crane, MD, MPH, S L. Gray, PharmD, MS, and E B. Larson, MD. "Risk of Dementia and AD with Prior Exposure to NSAIDs in an Elderly Community-Based Cohort." *Neurology* 72, no. 22 (June 2009): 1899–1905. doi: 10.1212/WNL.0b013e3181a18691
13. *Prescription Painkiller Overdoses in the US.* (2011, November 01). Retrieved May 23, 2016, from http://www.cdc.gov/Vital Signs/PainkillerOverdoses/index.html.
14. *Merck withdraws Vioxx Due to Heart Concerns.* (n.d.). Re trieved May 23, 2016, from http://money.cnn.com/2004/09/30/news/fortune500/merck/.
15. *Vioxx: This Pharmaceutical Drug Killed Over 60,000 People.* (n.d.). Retrieved May 23, 2016, from http://articles.mercola.com/sites/articles/archive/2012/05/14/mercks-adhd-drugs-unsafe.aspx.
16. Nesi, T. J. *Poison Pills: The Untold Story of the Vioxx Drug Scandal.* New York: Thomas Dunne Books, 2008.

17. Szalavitz, M. (n.d.). Merck | *Top 10 Drug Company Settlements* TIME.com. Retrieved May 23, 2016, from http://healthland.time.com/2012/09/17/pharma-behaving-badly-top-10-drug-company-settlements/slide/merck/.
18. Nadir, Arber, M.D., Craig J. Eagle, M.D., Julius Spicak, M.D., István Rácz, M.D., Petr Dite, M.D., Jan Hajer, M.D., Miroslav Zavoral, M.D., et. al. "Celecoxib for the Prevention of Colorectal Adenomatous Polyps for the PreSAP Trial Investigators." *New England Journal of Medicine* 355 (2006) :885-895. doi: 10.1056/NEJMoa061652.
19. Pfizer: (2012). Retrieved May 23, 2016, from http://www.hillmanfoundation.org/clearitwithsidney/pfizer-"they-swallowed-our-story-hook-line-and-sinker."
20. "Chronic Spinal Pain: A Randomized Clinical Trial Comparing Medication, Acupuncture, and Spinal Manipulation." *Spine* 28, no. 14 (July 2003): 1490-1500.
21. *Prescription Painkiller Overdoses in the US.* (2011, November 01). Retrieved May 23, 2016, from http://www.cdc.gov/VitalSigns/PainkillerOverdoses/index.html.
22. Brodke, Darrel S., MD, and Stephen M. Ritter, MD. "NonOperative Management of Low Back Pain and Lumbar Disc Degeneration." An Instructional Course Lecture, American Academy of Orthopedic Surgeons. *The Journal of Bone and Joint Surgery* 86-A No. 8, August 2004.
23. Studdert, David M., LL.B., Sc.D., M.P.H., Michelle M. Mello, J.D., Ph.D., M.Phil., and Troyen A. Brennan, M.D., J.D., M.P.H. "Financial Conflicts of Interest in Physicians' Relation ships with the Pharmaceutical Industry: Self-Regulation in

the Shadow of Federal Prosecution Legal Issues in Medicine." *The New England Journal of Medicine* (2004): 1891–1900.

24. Moynihan, R. "Who Pays for the Pizza? Redefining the Relationships Between Doctors and Drug Companies." 1: Entanglement. *BMJ 326*, no. 7400 (2003): 1189-1192. doi:10.1136/bmj.326.7400.1189.
25. *Docking the Tail That Wags the Dog: Banning Drug Reps from Academic Medical Facilities*, William B. Millard, PhD. Special Contributor to Annals News & Perspective Annals of Emergency Medicine. Vol 49 No 6 June 2007 785-791.
26. *Persuading the prescribers: pharmaceutical industry marketing and its influence on physicians and patients.* Fact Sheet November 11, 2013 http://www.pewtrusts.org/en/research-and-analysis/fact-sheets/2013/11/11/persuading-the-prescribers-pharmaceutical-industry-marketing-and-its-influence-on-physicians-and-patients.
27. *The medical profession and the pharmaceutical industry: When will we open our eyes?* Kerry J Breen, MB BS, MD, FRACP. The Medical Journal of Australia, April 19, 2004, 180 8 409-410.
28. *Generation Rx How Prescription Drugs Are Altering American Lives, Minds, and Bodies*, Greg Critser Houghton Mifflin Company 2005 Page 2.
29. *Record 4.02 Billion Prescriptions in 2011.* (n.d.). Retrieved May 23, 2016, from http://www.medicalnewstoday.com/releases/250213.php.
30. Paulette C. Morgan, "CRS Report for Congress," *Health Care Spending: Past trends and projections.* (2004).
31. Report: *Americans spent 8.5 percent more on prescription drugs in 2015.* (n.d.). Retrieved May 23, 2016, from

http://www.chicagotribune.com/business/ct-us-prescription-drug-spending-2015-20160414-story.html.

32. Mezei, I., Murinson, B.B., & Johns Hopkins Pain Curriculum Development Team. (2011). "Pain education in North American medical schools." *The Journal of Pain*, 12(12), 1199-1208.
33. Watt-Watson, J., McGillion, M., Hunter, J., Choiniere, M., Clark, A.J. Dewar, A., et al. (2009). A survey of prelicensure pain curricula in health science faculties in Canadian universities. *Pain Research & Management*, 14 (6), 439-444.
34. O'Rorke, J.E., Chen I., Genao, I., Panda, M., & Cykert, S. (2007). Physicians' comfort in caring for patients with chronic nonmalignant pain. *American Journal of Medical Sciences*, 333(2), 93-100.
35. Institute of Medicine, Committee on Advance Pain Research, Care, and Education. (2011). *Relieving pain in America: A blueprint for transforming prevention, care, education and research* (pp. 4-14) Publication copy. Washington, DC: National Academies Press.
36. Kolata, G. (2010). *Law May Do Little to Help Curb Unnecessary Care.* Retrieved April 28, 2016, from http://www.nytimes.com/2010/03/30/health/30use.html?_r=0.
37. Eisler, P., & Hansen, B. (2013). *Doctors perform thousands of unnecessary surgeries.* Retrieved April 28, 2016, from http://www.usatoday.com/story/news/nation/2013/06/18/unnecessary-surgery-usa-today-investigation/2435009/.
38. Waddell, Gordon. *The Back Pain Revolution.* Edinburgh: Churchill Livingstone, 1998
39. "Over-treating Chronic Back Pain: Time to back off?" *The Journal of the American Board of Family Medicine.* Vol. 22

Number 1, Jan 2009, pp 62-68 Richard Deyo, MD, Sohail Mirza, MD, Judith Turner, PhD, Brook Martin, MPH.

40. Iverson, T., Solberg, T.K., Romner, B., Wilsgaard, T., Twisk, J., Anke, A., et al. (2011). Effect of caudal epidural steroid or saline injection in chronic lumbar radiculopathy: Multicenter, blinded, randomized controlled trial. *British Medical Journa*l, 343, d5278.
41. Cohen, S.P. (2011). Epidural steroid injections for low back pain: Editorial. *British Medical Journal*, 343, d5301.
42. Ligament Injury and Healing: A Review of Current Clinical Diagnostics and Therapeutics, *The Open Rehabilitation Journal* 2013; No. 6; pp. 1-20, Russ A. Hauser MD, E.E. Dolan, H.J. Phillips, A.C. Newlin, R.E. Moore, B.A. Woldin.
43. *Benefits and Risks–Drug Pumps.* (n.d.). Retrieved May 24, 2016, from http://www.medtronic.com/patients/chronic-pain/device/drug-pumps/benefits-risks/index.htm.
44. Long-term Outcomes of Lumbar Fusion Among Workers' Compensation Subjects: A Historical Cohort Study. *Spine* 36 (4) pp320-332.
45. Martin BI, Mirza SK, Comstock BA et al. Reoperation rates following lumbar spine surgery and the influence of spinal fusion procedures. *Spine* 2007; 32:382-387.
46. Motion Compensation Associated with Single-Level Cervical Fusion: Where Does the Lost Motion Go? *Spine* Volume 31 (21) Oct 1, 2006 pp. 2439-2448, Schwab, John S., MSc; DiAngelo, Denis J., PhD; Foley, Kevin T. MD,
47. Keller RB, Atlas SJ, Soule DN, Singer DE, Deyo RA. Relations hip between rates and outcomes of operative treatment for

lumbar disc herniation and spinal stenosis. *Journal of Bone Joint Surgery* 1999; 81:752– 62.

48. Don and Caragee. Evidence-informed management of chronic low back pain with surgery. *The Spine Journal* 8. Pp. 114:120
49. *United States Trends and Regional Variations in Lumbar Spine Surgery: 1992–2003* James N. Weinstein, DO, MS; Jon D. Lurie, MD, MS; Patrick Olson, MD; Kristen K. Bronner, MS; Elliott S. Fisher, PhD; and Tamara S Morgan, MA.
50. *Most Frequent Operating Room Procedures Performed in U.S. Hospitals, 2003-2012* #186. Accessed October 29, 2016. https://www.hcup-us.ahrq.gov/reports/statbriefs/sb186-Operating-Room-Procedures-United-States-2012.jsp
51. *Spinal Fusions Serve as Case Study for Debate over When Cer tain Surgeries Are Necessary. Washington Post.* Accessed October 4, 2016. https://www.washingtonpost.com/business/economy/spinal-fusions-serve-as-case-study-for-debate-over-when-certain-surgeries-are-necessary/2013/10/27/5f015efa-25ff-11e3-b3e9-d97fb087acd6_story.html.
52. Carreyrou, John, and Tom Mcginty. *Top Spine Surgeons Reap Royalties, Medicare Bounty*. WSJ.com. December 20, 2010. Accessed October 04, 2016. wsj.com/articles.
53. KPCC, 89.3. *Selling the Spine: Doctors Profit in the OR, but at Whose Expense?* 89.3 KPCC. Accessed October 04, 2016. http://projects.scpr.org/longreads/selling-the-spine/.
54. Langevin, H. M., and K. J. Sherman. "Pathophysiological Model for Chronic Low Back Pain Integrating Connective Tissue and Nervous System Mechanisms." *Med Hypothesis* 68,

no. 1 (August 21, 2007): 74-80. Accessed October 18, 2016. https://www.ncbi.nlm.nih.gov/pubmed/16919887

55. Relief of fibromyalgia symptoms following discontinuation of dietary excitotoxins. Smith JD, Terpening, CM, Schmidt, SOF, Gums, JG. *The Annals of Pharmacotherapy*, June 2001, 35(6):702-6.
56. Institute of Medicine, Committee on Advance Pain Research, Care, and Education. (2011). *Relieving pain in America: A blueprint for transforming prevention, care, education and research* (pp. 4-14) Publication copy. Washington, DC: National Academies Press.
57. Vincent Y. Ma, BA; Leighton Chan, MD, MPH; Kadir J. Carruthers. BS. Incidence, Prevalence, Costs, and Impact on Disability of Common Conditions Requiring Rehabilitation in the United States: Stroke, Spinal Cord Injury, Traumatic Brain Injury, Multiple Sclerosis, Osteoarthritis, Rheumatoid Arthritis, Limb Loss, and Back Pain. *Archives of Physical Medicine and Rehabilitation* 2014; 95:986-95.
58. Institute of Medicine, Committee on Advance Pain Research, Care, and Education. (2011). *Relieving pain in America: A blueprint for transforming prevention, care, education and research* (pp. 4-14) Publication copy. Washington, DC: National Academies Press.
59. Systematic Literature Review of Imaging Features of Spinal Degeneration in Asymptomatic Population. W. Brinjikji, P. Luetmer, B. Comstock, B. Bresnahan, L. Chen, R. Deyo, S. Halabi, J. Turner, A. Avins, K. James, J. Wald, D. Kallmes, and J. Jarvik. *American Journal of Neuroradiology*, 2014.

60. Mayo Clinic Staff for Mayo Foundation for Medical Education and Research. *Growing Pains.* mayoclinic.org. Accessed 5/20/16Section 4.

Section 3

1. Taken from *In the Likeness of God* by Dr. Paul Brand and Philip Yancey Copyright © 2004 by Phillip Yancey. Use by permission of Zondervan. www.zondervan.com

Section 4

1. Chestnut, J.L. (2011). *The wellness & prevention paradigm.* Victoria, British Columbia, Canada: The Wellness Practice-Global Self Health. Pg. 185.
2. *Upright Radiology* Volume 63, Issue 9, September 2008, Pages 1035-1048 Clinical Radiology, F. Alyas, D. Connell, A. Saifuddin.
3. *The 14 Foundational Premises for the Scientific and Philosophical Validation of the Chiropractic Wellness Paradigm.* James Chestnut, B.Ed., M.Sc., D.C. Pg. 57.
4. A Theoretical Basis for Maintenance Spinal Manipulative Therapy, for the Chiropractic Profession *Journal of Chiropractic Humanities,* December 2011; Vol. 1; No. 1; pp.74-85 David N. Taylor DC, DACBN.
5. *The 14 Foundational Premises for the Scientific and Philosophical Validation of the Chiropractic Wellness Paradigm.* James Chestnut, B.Ed., M.Sc., D.C. pg. 225.

Section 5

1. *The Brain from Top to Bottom.* Accessed August 05, 2016. http://thebrain.mcgill.ca/flash/i/i_06/i_06_cr/i_06_cr_mou/i_06_cr_mou.html

2. Why Do Some Intervertebral Discs Degenerate, When Others (in the Same Spine) Do Not? *Clinical Anatomy* 2014, Michael A. Adams, Polly Lama, Uruj Zehra, Patricia Dolan, from the University of Bristol, UK.
3. Outcomes of Acute and Chronic Patients with Magnetic Resonance Imaging–Confirmed Symptomatic Lumbar Disc Herniations Receiving High Velocity, Low-Amplitude, Spinal Manipulative Therapy: A Prospective Observational Cohort Study with One-Year Follow-Up *Journal of Manipulative and Physiological Therapeutics* March/April 2014; Vol. 37; No. 3; pp. 155-163. Serafin Leemann, DC, Cynthia K. Peterson, RN, DC, MEd, Christof Schmid, DC, Bernard Anklin, DC, and B. Kim Humphreys, DC, PhDc. The authors are from Zurich, Switzerland.
4. James Chestnut, B. E. (2003). *The 14 Foundational Premises for the Scientific and Philosophical Validation of the Chiropractic Wellness Paradigm*. Victoria, British Columbia: The Well ness Practice–Global Self Health Corp, pg 51.
5. *Treatment of Lumbar Intervertebral Disc Protrusions by Manipulation Clinical Orthopedics and Related Research* February 1987, pp. 47-55 Paul Pang-Fu Kuo and Zhen-Chao Loh from the Department of Orthopedic Surgery, Shanghai Second Medical College, and Chief Surgeon, Department of Orthopedic Surgery, Rui Jin Hospital, Shanghai, China.
6. James Chestnut, B. E. (2003). *The 14 Foundational Premises for the Scientific and Philosophical Validation of the Chiropractic Wellness Paradigm*. Victoria, British Columbia: The Well ness Practice–Global Self Health Corp.

7. Dr. James Chestnus B.Ed., M. D. (n.d.). *Chiropractic or Chiropractic plus Prescription Drugs?* http://chiropracticsocietywi.org/save-chiropractic/.
8. James Chestnut, B. E. (2003). *The 14 Foundational Premises for the Scientific and Philosophical Validation of the Chiropractic Wellness Paradigm.* Victoria, British Columbia: The Wellness Practice–Global Self Health Corp.
9. Long-Term Follow-up of a Randomized Clinical Trial Assessing the Efficacy of Medication, Acupuncture, and Spinal Ma nipulation for Chronic Mechanical Spinal Pain Syndromes, *Journal of Manipulative and Physiological Therapeutics* January 2005, Volume 28, Number 1 Reinhold Muller, PhD, Lynton G.F. Giles, DC, PhD.
10. Giles LGF, Muller R. Chronic spinal pain: a randomized clinical trial comparing medication, acupuncture and spinal manipulation, *Spine* 2003; 28:1490-1503 *Spine*, July 15, 2003; 28(14): 1490-1502
11. Bronfort et al. (2008) Evidence-informed management of chronic low back pain with spinal manipulation and mobilization. *The Spine Journal* 8 213-225.
12. Spinal Manipulation, Medication, or Home Exercise with Advice for Acute and Subacute Neck Pain: A Randomized Trial *Annals of Internal Medicine* January 3, 2012; Vol. 156; pp. 1-10 Gert Bronfort, DC, PhD; Roni Evans, DC, MS; Alfred V. Anderson, DC, MD; Kenneth H. Svendsen, MS; Yiscah Bracha, MS; and Richard H. Grimm, MD, MPH, PhD.
13. Spinal manipulation compared with back school and with in dividually delivered physiotherapy for the treatment of chronic low back pain: A randomized trial with one-year fol-

low-up. *Clinical Rehabilitation* January 2010; Vol. 24, No. 1; pp.26-36 Francesca Cecchi, Raffaello Molino-Lova, Massimiliano Chiti, Guido Pasquini, Anita Paperini: The authors are from the University of Florence, Italy.

14. Health Maintenance Care in Work-Related Low Back Pain and Its Association with Disability Recurrence, *Journal of Occupational and Environmental Medicine* March 14, 2011; Vol. 197 [epub] Manuel Cifuentes, MD, PhD, Joanna Willetts, MS, Radoslaw Wasiak, PhD, MA, MS.
15. Johnson, DC, Kurtz Z, ME (2001). Diminished use of osteopathic manipulative therapy and its impact on the uniqueness of the osteopathic profession. *Acad Med* 76 (8): 821-8].
16. Chiropractors and Low Back Pain, *The Lancet* July 28, 1990, p. 220 The editors review the June 2, 1990 *British Medical Journal* article by Meade, Low back pain of mechanical origin: randomized comparison of chiropractic and hospital outpatient treatment.
17. Effects of Early Motion on Healing of Musculoskeletal Tissues, *Hand Clinics* Volume 12, Number 1, February 1996, Joseph Buckwalter, MD, from the Department of Orthopedics, University of Iowa.
18. Balthazard, Pierre, Pierre de Goumoens, Gilles Rivier, Philippe Demeulenaere, Pierluigi Ballabeni, and Olivier Dériaz. Manual therapy followed by specific active exercises versus a placebo followed by specific active exercises on the improvement of functional disability in patients with chronic nonspecific low back pain: a randomized controlled trial, Bio Med Central (BMC) *Musculoskeletal Disorders* 2012 13:162

19. Ingeborg B C Korthals-de Bos, Jan L Hoving, Maurits W van Tulder, Maureen P M H Rutten-van Mölken, Herman J Adèr, Henrica C W de Vet, Bart W Koes, Hindrik Vondeling, Lex M Bouter. Cost effectiveness of physiotherapy, manual therapy, and general practitioner care for neck pain: economic evaluation alongside a randomized controlled trial *British Medical Journal*; 326:911; April 26, 2003
20. Hoving, Jan Lucas, PT, PhD; Bart W. Koes, PhD; Henrica C.W. de Vet, PhD; Danielle A.W.M. van der Windt, PhD; Willem J.J. Assendelft, MD, PhD; Henk van Mameren, MD, PhD; Walter L.J.M. Devillé, MD, PhD; Jan J.M. Pool, PT; Rob J.P.M Scholten, MD, PhD; and Lex M. Bouter, Ph.D. Manual Therapy, Physical Therapy, or Continued Care by a General Practioner for Patients with Neck Pain *Annals of Internal Medicine* 136, No. 10, (2002): 713-722 May 21, 2002
21. Ingeborg B C; Korthals-de Bos, Jan L Hoving, Maurits W van Tulder, Maureen P M H Rutten-van Mölken, Herman J Adèr, Henrica C W de Vet, Bart W Koes, Hindrik Vondeling, and Lex M Bouter. "Cost effectiveness of physiotherapy, manual therapy, and general practitioner care for neck pain: economic evaluation alongside a randomized controlled trial," *British Medical Journal* 326, no. 911, April 26, 2003.
22. Lindstrom, I., Ohlund, C., Eek C., Wallin, L., Peterson, L. E., Fordyce, W. E., et al (1992). The effect of graded activity on patients with subacute low back pain: a randomized prospective clinical study with an operant-condition behavioral approach [Abstract]. *Physical Therapy*, 72 (4) 279-290.
23. Taimela, S., Diederich, C., Hubsch, M., & Heinricy, M. (2000). The role of physical exercise and inactivity in pain recurrence

and absenteeism from work after active outpatient rehabilit= ation for recurrent or chronic low back pain: A follow-up study. *Spine*, 25 (14), 1809-1816.

24. Kool, J., de Bie, R., Oesch, P., Knusle, O., van den Brandt, P., & Bachman, S. (2004) Exercise reduces sick leave in patients with non-acute non-specific low back pain: A meta-analysis. *Journal of Rehabilitation Medicine*, 36 (2), 49-62.
25. Maul, I., Laubli, T., Oliveri, M., & Krueger, H. Long-term effects of supervised physical training in secondary prevention of low back pain. *European Spine Journal*, 14 (6), 599-611.
26. Choi, B.K.L., Verbeek, J.H., Tam, W. W-S., & Jiang, J.Y. (2010). Exercises for the prevention of recurrences of low-back pain. *Occupational and Environmental Medicine*, 67, 795-796.
27. Sofi, F., Molino, L. R., Nucida, V., Taviani, A., Benvenuti, F., Stuart, M., et al. (2011) Adaptive physical therapy and back pain: A non-randomized community-based intervention trial. European *Journal of Physical and Rehabilitative Medicine*, 47 (4), 543-549.
28. Hayden, J., van Tulder, M.W., Mlmivaara, A., & Koes, B.W. (2005). Exercise therapy for treatment of non-specific low back pain. *Cochrane Database of Systematic Reviews*, 2005 (3), CD000335.
29. Hides, JA; Richardson, CA; Jull, GA. Multifidus muscle recovery is not automatic after resolution of acute, first-episode of low back pain. *Spine* 1996; 21 (23): 2763-2769.
30. Hayden, J.A., van Tulder, M.W., Malmivarra, A., & Koes, B.W. (2005). Meta-analysis: Exercise therapy for nonspecific low back pain [Abstract]. *Annals of Internal Medicine*, 142 (9), 765-775.

31. Walach, H., Güthlin, C., König, M. (2003). Efficacy of massage therapy in chronic pain: a pragmatic randomized trial. J Altern *Complement Med.* 9(6), 837-46.

32. Seers, K., Crichton, N., Martin, J., Coulson, K., Carroll, D. (2008). A randomized controlled trial to assess the effective ness of a single session of nurse administered massage for short term relief of chronic non-malignant pain. *BMC Nurs.* 7, 10.

33. Frey Law, L.A., Evans, S., Knudtson, J. Nus, S., Scholl, K., Sluka, K.A. (2008). Massage reduces pain perception and hy peralgesia in experimental muscle pain: a randomized, con trolled trial. *J Pain.* 9(8), 714-21.

34. Moraska, A., Chandler, C., Edmiston-Schaetzel, A., Franklin, G., Calenda, E.L., Enebo, B. (2008). *Comparison of a targeted and general massage protocol on strength, function, and symptoms associated with carpal tunnel syndrome: a randomized pilot study.* J Altern.

35. Quinn C., Chandler C., Moraska A. Massage Therapy and Fre quency of Chronic Tension Headaches. *American Journal of Public Health* 92(10); 1657-61; Oct 2002.

36. Chou, R., & Huffman, L.H. (2007). Non-pharmacologic therapies for acute and chronic low back pain: A review of the evidence for an American Pain Society/American College of Physicians clinical practice guidelines. *Annals of Internal Medicine,* 147 (7), 492-504.

37. Non-operative Management of Low Back Pain and Lumbar Disc Degeneration: An Instructional Course Lecture, American Academy of Orthopaedic Surgeons. *The Journal of Bone*

and Joint Surgery, Vol. 86-A, Number 8, August 2004. Darrell S. Brodke, MD, and Stephen M. Ritter, MD.

38. Eberhard Lang, K. L. (n.d.). Multidisciplinary rehabilitation versus usual care for chronic low back pain in the community: effects on quality of life. *Spine Journal,* pp. DOI: http://dx.doi.org/10.1016/S1529-9430(03)00028-7.
39. Heymans MW1, v. T. (2005, Oct 1). Back schools for nonspecific low back pain: a systematic review within the framework of the Cochrane Collaboration Back Review Group. *Spine,* pp. 2153-2163.
40. Koes BW, v. T. (1994, Aug). The efficacy of back schools: a review of randomized clincal trials. *Journal of Clinical Epidemiology,* pp. 47 (8): 851-62.
41. Lønn, J. H., Glomsrød, B. P., Soukup, M. G., Bø, K. P., & Larsen, S. M. (1999, May 1). Active Back School: Prophylactic Management for Low Back Pain: A Randomized, Controlled, 1-Year Follow-Up Study. *Spine,* pp. 865-871.
42. RP, D. F. (1995). Efficacy of comprehensive rehabilitation programs and back school for patients with low back pain. *Physical Therapy.,* pp. 75 (10): 865-78.
43. Tavafian SS, J. A. (2008, Jul 1). A randomized study of back school with patients with low back pain: quality of life at three, six, nine, and twelve months. *Spine,* pp. 1617-1625.
44. Sedigheh Sadat Tavafian1, A. J. (2007, Feb 28). Low back pain education and short term quality of life: a radomized trial. *BMC Musculoskeletal Disorders,* p. 8:21.
45. Van Tulder MW, E. R. (2000). B*ack schools for non-specific low back pain.* Cochrane Database Syst Rev, p. (2): CD000261.

46. Roger Chou, M. F. (2016, February). *Noninvasive Treatments for Low Back Pain.* Effective Health Care Program.
47. The Efficacy of Manual Treatment in Low-back Pain: A Clinical Trial. Arkuszewski Z. *Manual Medicine*, 1986;2;68-71.
48. A Randomized Trial of Manipulation for Low-back Pain in a Medical Setting. Godfrey CM., et al. *Spine*,1984; 9:301-304.
49. Goertz, Christine M. DC, PhD; Cynthia R. Long, PhD, Maria A. Hondras, DC, MPH; Richard Petri, MD; Roxana Delgado, MS; Dana J. Lawrence, DC; Edward F. Owens, MS, DC; William C. Meeker, DC, MPH. "Adding Chiropractic Manipulative Therapy to Standard Medical Care for Patients with Acute Low Back Pain: Results of a Pragmatic Randomized Comparative Effectiveness Study," *Spine* 38, no. 8 (2013): 627–634.
50. Furlan, A., M. Imamura, M, T. Dryden, and E. Irvin, (2008). Massage for low back pain. Cochran Database of Systematic Reviews, 2008 (4), CD001929Cherkin, D.C., Sherman, K.J., Kahn, J., Wellman, R., Cook, A., J., Johnson, E., et al. (2011). A comparison of the effects of 2 types of massage and usual care on chronic low back pain. *Annals of Internal Medicine*, 155(1), 1-9.
51. Cherkin, D.C., Sherman, K.J., Kahn, J., Wellman, R., Cook, A., J., Johnson, E., et al. (2011). A comparison of the effects of 2 types of massage and usual care on chronic low back pain. *Annals of Internal Medicine*, 155(1), 1-9.
52. United Kingdom back pain exercise and manipulation (UK BEAM) randomized trial: cost effectiveness of physical treat ments for back pain in primary care, UK BEAM Trial Team

(Andrea Manca), *British Medical Journal* 2004; 329:1381, December11, 2004.

53. Espi-Lopez., GV; Zurriaga-Llorens, R.; Monzani, L. Falla "The effect of manipulation plus massage therapy versus massage therapy alone in people with tension-type headache. A randomized controlled clinical trial." *European Journal of Physical Rehabilitation Medicine,* Mar 18, 2016.
54. Efficacy of comprehensive rehabilitation programs and back school for patients with low back pain: a meta-analysis. *Physical Therapy*. 1995; 75(10):865-78 (ISSN: 0031-9023) Di Fabio RP.
55. *A Randomized, Controlled Trial of Manual Therapy and Specific Adjuvant Exercise for Chronic Low Back Pain*, Michael E. Geisser, Ph.D., Elizabeth A. Wiggert, P.T., Andrew J. Haig, M.D., and Miles O. Colwell, M.D.
56. Cuesta-Vargas, Al, J. C. Garcia-Romero, M. Arroyo-Morales, A.M. Diego-Acosta, AM, and D. J. Daly. Exercise, manual ther apy, and education with or without high intensity deep-water running for nonspecific chronic low back pain: a pragmatic randomized controlled trial. *American Journal of Physical Med-Rehabilitation,* 2011 Jul; 90(7):526-34; quiz 538-8. Doi:10.1097/PHM.0b013e21821a71d0,
57. Troyanovich. et al. Structural Rehabilitation of the spine and posture: Rationale for treatment beyond resolution of symptoms. *JMPT* 1998.
58. *Effects of Early Motion on Healing of Musculoskeletal Tissues, Hand Clinics.* Volume 12, Number 1, February 1996, Joseph Buckwalter, MD from the Department of Orthopedics, University of Iowa.

59. Hauser, Russ A., MD, E.E. Dolan, H.J. Phillips, A.C. Newlin, R.E. Moore, and B.A. Woldin "Ligament Injury and Healing: A Review of Current Clinical Diagnostics and Therapeutics," *The Open Rehabilitation Journal,* 2013; No. 6; pp. 1-20.
60. Peterson, C., C. Schmidt , S. Leemann, B. Anklin, and B. Humphreys. Outcomes from Magnetic Resonance Imaging: Confirmed Symptomatic Cervical Disk Herniation Patient Treated with High-Velocity, Low-Amplitude Spinal Manipulation Therapy: A Prospective Cohort Study with Three-Month Follow Up, *JMT* Oct. 2013; Vol. 36; pp. 461-467
61. Spinal Manipulation in the Treatment of Low Back Pain, *Canadian Family Physician,* March 1985, Vol. 31, pp. 535-540W. H. Kirkaldy-Willis and J. D. Cassidy. Dr. Kirkaldy-Willis is a Professor Emeritus of Orthopedics and director of the Low Back Pain Clinic at the University Hospital, Saskatoon, Canada.
62. Hall, H., Conservative Management of Low Back Pain, excerpt in *Medicine North America,* Oct. 26,1988, 4878-4885.
63. Jenna & Machaly (2011) Does Maintained Spinal Manipulation Therapy for Chronic Nonspecific Low Back Pain Result in Better Long-Term Outcome? *Spine* 36 (18) 1427-37
64. A theoretical basis for maintenance spinal manipulative therapy for the chiropractic profession, *Journal of Chiropractic Humanities*, December 2011; Vol. 1; No. 1; pp.74-85 David N. Taylor, DC, DACBN.
65. Alcantra et al. Chiropractic Management of a patient with myasthenia gravis and vertebral subluxations *JMPT* 1999; 22 (5).

66. Scar Formation and Ligament Healing [Surgical Biology for the Clinician], *Canadian Journal of Surgery*, December 1998; Vol. 41; No. 6; pp. 425-429, Kevin Hildebrand, MD and Cyril Frank, MD.

67. McGill, S. Stability: from biomechanical concept to chiropractic practice. *JCCA* 1999; 43 (2).

68. Maroon, JC, Bost, JW; *Omega-3 fatty acids (fish oil) as an anti-inflammatory: an alternative to nonsteroidal anti-inflammatory drugs for discogenic pain;* April 2006;65(4); pp. 326-31.

69. *How Much Omega Sufficiency® Is Required Each Day? Innate Choice.* Accessed September 27, 2016. http://innatechoice.com/viewfaq.cfm?id=20AB76E3-A5E5-6F58-274971E9A12C47C.

70. Al Faraj, Al Mutairl K. Vitamin D and Chronic Low Back Pain in Saudi Arabia, *Spine* 2003; 28;172-179.

71. *Innate Choice.* Accessed September 27, 2016. http://innatechoice.com/viewfaq.cfm?id=63A4E756-E2E9-7E2B-17F3347806D92AE2

Made in the USA
Middletown, DE
04 September 2022

73183613R00156